# YOUR BACK
# YOUR HEALTH

Dr Paul Sherwood, consultant in physical medicine (treatment using massage, manipulation, electrical and other equipment), trained at Cambridge University and the Westminster Hospital. After achieving a degree in medicine he worked as a house surgeon at Westminster Hospital, and later at Barts before becoming a consultant at a number of hospitals. He has been developing his own form of physical medicine at his private clinic in London over a period of 40 years.

Dr Sherwood is the author of *Asthma and Beyond*, *The Heart Revolution* and *Get Well, Stay Well*.

Dr Sherwood's Practice
2 Devonshire Place
London W1G 6HJ

Telephone 020 7580 4691
Fax 020 7224 2832

Email: mail@DrSherwood.co.uk

www.DrSherwood.co.uk

www.YourBackYourHealth.co.uk

The Back and Beyond
The Heart Revolution
Get Well, Stay Well

# YOUR BACK
# YOUR HEALTH

DR PAUL SHERWOOD

arrow books

Published by Arrow Books in 2004

1 3 5 7 9 10 8 6 4 2

Copyright © Dr Paul Sherwood 2004

Dr Paul Sherwood has asserted his right under the Copyright, Designs and
Patents Act, 1988, to be identified as the author of this work

Arrow Books Limited
The Random House Group Limited
20 Vauxhall Bridge Road, London SW1V 2SA

Random House Australia (Py) Limited
20 Alfred Street, Milsons Point, Sydney,
New South Wales 2061, Australia

Random House New Zealand Limited
18 Poland Road, Glenfield,
Auckland 10, New Zealand

Random House South Africa (Pty) Limited
Endulini, 5A Jubilee Road, Parktown 2193, South Africa

The Random House Group Limited Reg. No. 954009

www.randomhouse.co.uk

A CIP catalogue record for this book is available from the British Library

Papers used by Random House UK are natural, recyclable products
made from wood grown in sustainable forests. The manufacturing processes conform
to the environmental regulations of the country of origin

ISBN 0 09 946802 6

Typeset by SX Composing DTP, Rayleigh, Essex
Printed and bound in Great Britain by
Biddles Ltd, Guildford and Kings Lynn

To my much-loved family Robin, Julian and Amanda
and my granddaughters Emily and Juliet Kitson

# CONTENTS

Foreword by Dr Brian Bradnock    ix

Author's Note    xi

Acknowledgements    xiii

Introduction    xv

1    Know Your Back    1
     The anatomy and function of your spinal column

2    Your Painful Back    19
     The cause of recurrent chronic back pain

3    Your Back in Question    43
     Clear answers to common queries

4    Back to Specifics    65
     Identifying pain associated with your back

5    Your Back and a Healthy Sex Life    85
     A good reason to have effective treatment for your back

6    Back to Front    95
     Your back problem and a common new disease

7    Your Back and ME    114
     Why ME is not such a mysterious disease

8    Taking Your Back Seriously    136
     Your back as an unsuspected cause of other diseases

9    Heart Problems and Your Back    176
     A new concept in the cause and treatment of coronary thrombosis

10   Back to Good Health    217
     Treatment for your back problem

Appendix I Description of treatment
A note for your therapist    249
Appendix II Action plan for immediate relief of back pain    263
Appendix III Daily five-minute exercise plan    266
Appendix IV Resuscitation    270
Appendix V A note on tonsillectomy by Mike Dilkes MS, FRCS(Ed), FRCS(Otol), FRCS(ORL)    277

Glossary    280
Useful addresses    290
Index    293

# FOREWORD

I have used Doctor Sherwood's regime, over the past ten years, in the treatment of back pain and to treat patients suffering from chronic fatigue syndrome. Many patients have been transformed and have returned to live normal lives.

Dr Sherwood's ideas on the causation and treatment of back pain will surely revolutionise modern day treatment.

Brian Bradnock FRCSEd, FRCSOrth
Consultant Orthopaedic Surgeon
St Albans City Hospital
Hertfordshire
England

# AUTHOR'S NOTE

This book is concerned with non-specific back pain, that is pain that cannot be attributed to a specific disease. It is important that all back problems be given a proper medical assessment to eliminate all diagnosable causes. It is only after full investigation that a verdict of non-specific back pain can be reached.

I must stress that my recommended treatment is always given alongside, not instead of, other medical care. All back sufferers should seek medical advice and help, especially for the complications that can occur.

The various secondary effects of back trouble, such as peptic ulcer or arthritic joints, should also be medically supervised. These conditions may give rise to serious complications and it is important that you continue to be supervised by your own doctor or specialist during treatment to the back. The secondary illness will usually clear up within a few weeks of treatment to the back but it makes sense to attack the problem on all fronts, especially if the symptoms are bad.

As far as the chapter on heart problems is concerned, this applies only to those people who have recovered from heart attacks or have never had one. It is in no way intended to replace or modify the orthodox medical treatment of a heart attack itself.

# ACKNOWLEDGEMENTS

To Caroline Shott who threatened death if this book was not written and to my family and friends who made my life unbearable when I was not getting on with my work. Thanks are also due to Anne and Robin Wilson who provided me with a palm tree to sit under beside their swimming pool in the South of France, so that I could type the manuscript in (relative) peace and quiet.

A special acknowledgement must go to Laura Garcia who went through the original book and suggested many of the changes and improvements that have been incorporated.

I would also like to give especial thanks to Marion Paull, the editor, who has honed the book into a readable form and ironed out all the mistakes.

# INTRODUCTION

⸙ But doctor, I only leaned forward to look in the mirror. I wanted to see if I had a pimple on my chin. The next thing I knew my back became agonizingly painful and I haven't been able to move for three days. ⸙

⸙ I am hoping you can do something. For the last six years I've had acute attacks of back pain and have been off work for three or four days each time. ⸙

⸙ If I do anything – carry the shopping, a little work in the garden or, worst of all, lift up my three-year-old daughter – I get pain in my back within twenty-four hours. It's spoiling my life. ⸙

These are common complaints from people coming to me for consultation. Most say their GPs could not help. Some back-pain sufferers are told that the pain is all in the mind, the young are reassured that they have growing pains, older patients are told that they must expect back trouble with their advancing years and others that they must simply learn to live with it.

People who suffer from non-specific back pain, that is pain that is not the result of a specific disease, have to live with aches that may restrict their activities. Some try to find their own temporary solutions for coping with the pain by swimming, taking up yoga or self-manipulation but they live with the fear of the next attack and, on the whole, have little positive help from the medical profession. For a heart attack, most people trust their specialist's expertise and are confident that they are receiving the best possible care. Is it not strange that back troubles take people to the large army of alternative practitioners more often than to medical consultants?

Unhappy with the advice and treatment offered by their doctors, many back-pain sufferers try osteopathy, relaxation techniques, chiropratic, acupuncture or faith healing, any or all of which may provide immediate relief. Osteopaths, chiropractors and others are able to help, rapidly and painlessly, patients who were previously confined to bed, required to wear a corset or collar, or to undergo surgery. Indeed, it is doubtful if their treatment of acute pain could be bettered (acute meaning arising suddenly and of short duration). It is only in the long-term that these treatments may not prove to be so successful. Most people find that their back problems recur but there is, however, much to be learned from the less orthodox practitioners.

I go to an osteopath or chiropractor each time my back "goes out". For a number of years they have kept me going but now that treatment doesn't seem to stop the pain coming back. What I want is permanent relief.

I have been going to an osteopath for twelve years for each attack of pain and have always been satisfied. But on this last occasion he could not help. What else can I do?

## TAKING THE PROBLEM SERIOUSLY

Back trouble needs to be taken a great deal more seriously than most people, including *many* in the medical profession, believe. Intermittent back pain is debilitating and – as many alternative practitioners know – a person with a bad back often suffers from a number of associated conditions, such as tiredness and headaches. These are very often helped by successful treatment to the back.

More than that, I have come to the conclusion that many complaints, including ME (myalgic encephalomyelitis, or post-viral syndrome, sometimes called chronic fatigue syndrome), migraine, indigestion and even stomach and duodenal ulcers are often caused by back problems. By treating the root cause in the back, these complaints can usually be cured.

In the course of my 50 years' research and practice, I have come across a common condition characterized by tiredness, depression, a tensed-up feeling, indigestion and aches between the shoulders. This so far unrecognized disease, which I have called HST (hypo-sympathetic tone), is making life a misery for many thousands of people. It is caused by back trouble and with a correct diagnosis is as easy to treat as the back itself.

My approach to back trouble is holistic. I work in the belief that all parts of the body are connected and interrelated. Unlike those in the medical profession who concentrate on one organ and all the different problems associated with that one part, I concentrate on a *family* of illnesses and whichever part of the body it assails. The orthodox medical principles of my theory are not new but I believe that my reassessment of how they are put together has never been advocated before.

The Back Pain Association estimates that every year over three million Britons consult a family doctor because of back trouble. For well over half these sufferers there is little positive help. They are told that their pain can only be relieved when they suffer a new attack. If the pain goes away, they are told that they are cured of their trouble – until it happens again. I do not agree with this approach. I believe that patients with back pain can be offered immediate relief *and* be prevented from having recurring bouts – if they are given the correct treatment.

## THE UNDERLYING PROBLEM

Very many people are confused because their symptoms do not seem to match the explanation, and treatment often makes them feel worse. Their pain puzzles them. Why is it so often worse in the morning after a night's rest, or after considerable exercise? Why do they feel so much better in sunny weather? There are logical explanations for these and many other seeming paradoxes.

Contrary to popular opinion, back pain is not an inevitable part of old age, and poor posture is not to blame for back trouble. Bed rest has few benefits, surgery is only ever necessary in extreme cases, traction and corsets often make the problem worse and anti-inflammatory drugs all too often have little effect. Alternative practitioners offer positive help but this is usually only short-term and does little to relieve the underlying problem.

So, you might ask, how is my theory and form of treatment so different? The crux of it lies in the fact that the majority of back-pain therapists concentrate on relieving the *present* attack of pain but do little to stop *future* attacks. I believe that we should be looking beyond the actual attack of pain to the deep-rooted cause. When a patient has intermittent back pain the basic problem is present all the time. The pain is a result of a change in the underlying problem; by ridding the patient of pain the therapist isn't necessarily doing anything to correct the basic problem.

I believe that all non-specific back pain has its root in an old injury, caused by a fall, perhaps, or some hard jolt or twist that disturbed the spinal column. The back may remain symptomless for years. Often a minor episode, such as leaning over the bar or reaching to pick up a cup, may spark off trouble. The pain may come and go over the years but the basic trouble remains, as do the symptoms of the other complaints already mentioned.

My work over the past 50 years has shown that by promoting the recovery of bruised facet joints in the spine, it is possible for a troublesome back to be permanently restored to good health. The tools and techniques of my treatment are widely available in physiotherapy departments all over the country – manipulation, remobilization, massage, ultrasonic waves and surged faradism, (which is a controlled electrical current designed to stimulate the muscle). By using this physical medicine to treat the cause rather than the symptoms, I have given most of my patients long-lasting relief from both back pain and the associated illnesses, and there is no risk involved.

## EFFECTIVE TREATMENT

There is some confusion between what is meant by treatment and the means by which it is carried out. Patients have often told me that they have had manipulation, for instance, in the past and that it helped temporarily only, so they dismissed it as being of little value. In fact, manipulation, ultrasonic waves and the other techniques are simply tools to carry out the treatment and are not the treatment itself. It is important to understand this distinction.

Let us suppose a bearing keeps wearing out in a car engine. The repair is to replace the bearing, and spanners and screwdrivers are the tools the garage uses to carry out the repair. If each new bearing also rapidly wears out, you may well go to another garage for a second opinion. At this garage the mechanic may say that the real problem is a blocked oil filter, which needs replacing. He will use spanners and screwdrivers and, once the oil filter is renewed, the car works perfectly and you have no further trouble.

The mechanic at the second garage used the same tools as at the first but with greater success. By discovering the underlying trouble in the blocked oil filter he could put the tools to more effective use and provide permanent repair. Ultrasonic waves, massage and manipulation are equivalent to the spanners and screwdrivers used by the mechanic and similarly they can be used for different purposes with varying degrees of success. By treating the basic cause of back pain, just as the mechanic at the second garage worked on the underlying problem with the car, it is possible to help back problems to a great extent using techniques and instruments that are widely available.

In Britain, around 80 million working days are lost each year through back pain and the figure is rising. Those days cost the economy around three billion pounds in 1992. On its own the amount is shocking, but think of the days lost through related illnesses. One of these may be heart disease – 35 million working days lost each year.

How many more millions of pounds are lost through lack of effective diagnosis and treatment for back pain? In Britain alone, there is a cost of over £350 million to the health service to treat these patients, plus £70 million for heart patients. The treatment I suggest, which is outlined in chapter 10 and Appendix 1, could save the health service millions of pounds per year. Use it as a basis for seeking help through your own doctor or from a suitably trained physiotherapist, osteopath or other therapist in your area.

Back trouble can have serious repercussions throughout the whole body and I hope this book will make doctors give the problem a major rethink and encourage debate among the medical profession as well as the general public.

The scale of devastation caused by coronary heart disease in Britain alone is tremendous and it continues despite the efforts of the world's medical practitioners. Without doubt, heart research has achieved many successes. The knowledge the medical profession has acquired concerning both prevention and treatment is one of the miracles of modern times. However, heart disease is still Britain's biggest killer and disabler, and researchers are still looking for clues to many outstanding anomalies. It is because of this that I feel justified in putting forward my ideas of diagnosis and treatment, related to the back, in the hope that they may help diminish the appalling figures.

There are many theories about the cause and relief of back pain, and while mine might seem to be just one of the many, it has produced an effective treatment that has already helped thousands of people. Almost everyone who suffers from non-specific back pain can be completely cured with the correct tools and diagnosis.

## ON A PERSONAL NOTE

I can fully sympathize when back-pain sufferers become impatient. In my younger days, I had a bout of back trouble. It began as pins and needles in my leg and progressed until I sporadically lost the use of the leg completely. At the same time I was suffering a lot of pain in my back. Like so many others, I was referred from one practitioner to another. Neurological, orthopaedic and physical medicine specialists all offered different diagnoses and suggested different treatments.

After a year or two of unsuccessful treatment, I was getting most frustrated with the situation and couldn't help saying on several occasions, 'Surely, someone must be able to help me.' I did everything the various specialists told me to do, even enduring bed rest for a whole month. Osteopathy helped a great deal but each time the relief was temporary. Traction made it worse. Nothing seemed to offer any effective help. When surgery was recommended, I decided that enough was enough.

Having already spent some time treating patients with non-specific back pain, I was convinced that the original cause of my problem was a fall down the stairs during a holiday a few years before. So, I asked a GP friend to train with me for a few weeks and then asked him to work on my back using my directions. Within three months, I had made a full recovery.

Over the years, I have found that many patients who consult me have, like me, already had several years of appointments and disappointments. 'I have tried everything and now I've been told that I must learn to live with the pain and inconvenience. Is there anything else?' is the common cry for help. In answer, this book describes a treatment that I have been developing for 50 years, which offers reasonably permanent relief not only for back pain but also for associated problems.

# 1 KNOW YOUR BACK

## The anatomy and function of your spinal column

If you are to understand back pain and its related problems, it is important to have some knowledge of how the spine works and the part it plays within the body machine. So, with the help of diagrams, let us consider briefly the anatomy and functions of the spinal column.

## THE SPINAL COLUMN

The spine has three important functions:

- **Support**. As you can see from figure 1.1 on page 2, the spine is an extension of the legs, supporting the whole of the abdomen and thorax (the area between the abdomen and neck) and providing a firm base for the weight of the head. It acts like a frame, connected to all the soft tissues and bones from the legs, the pelvis, the arms, the head and the ribs.

- **Protection**. The spinal column works in association with the ribs to give a measure of protection to the heart and lungs, and with the pelvis to protect the lower abdominal organs. Much more importantly, it also encloses the spinal cord. This vital and vulnerable structure of spinal nerves runs from the brain stem down

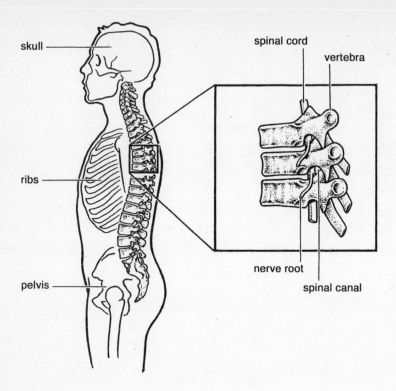

*Figure 1.1* The spine is the centre of support, protecting the spinal cord and – with the ribs, skull and pelvis – the brain, heart, lungs and abdomen. In the inset, note how the spinal cord runs up through the spinal canal in the vertebrae.

to the top of the lumbar spine (the part of the spine located between the lowest ribs and the hip bones), where it divides into smaller nerves known as the cauda equina.

- **Mobility**. The third function is to allow some movement of the trunk, making it possible to bend backwards, forwards and sideways, and to rotate. This means the body can move on the pelvis and the head can move independently from the rest of the trunk (see figure 1.2 on page 3).

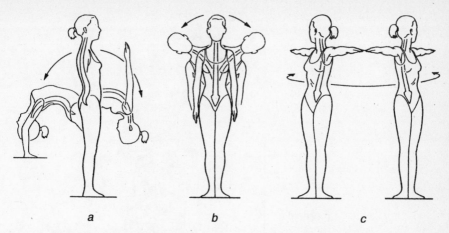

*Figure 1.2* for such a strong structure, the spine is enormously flexible, allowing movement: backwards, and forwards (*a*), side to side (*b*), and rotationally (*c*).

## STRUCTURE

The spinal column has a gentle S-shape. The curve is flexible and capable of sudden alteration. By absorbing the force of unexpected shocks or blows, it provides a valuable cushioning effect.

### Vertebrae

The spine is made up of 29 small bones called vertebrae, placed one on top of another. Each individual vertebra is shaped rather like a small tin of food, round with a flat top and bottom. Most of the vertebrae are separate but five near the bottom are fused into one single bone known as the sacrum. At this point in the spinal column rigidity and strength are more important than flexibility. At the extreme end of the spine is our residual tail called the coccyx, which is made up of a number of small jointed bones (see figure 1.3).

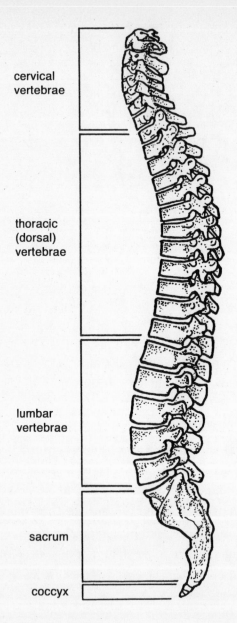

cervical
vertebrae

thoracic
(dorsal)
vertebrae

lumbar
vertebrae

sacrum

coccyx

*Figure 1.3* These are the divisions of the spine. It's important to indentify which vertebrae are affected before treatment can be undertaken.

## Intervertebral discs

The vertebrae are separated from each other by intervertebral discs, which are shaped like old-fashioned pillboxes. Each disc is a sort of thick fibrous box, which is welded to the vertebra above and the one below. The discs are filled with an elastic jelly and it is this that gives the spinal column its flexibility.

Without these discs the movement of the spine would be very limited. Picture the spinal column as a pile of food tins. Try stacking a few tins on top of one another and you will find that with two hard flat surfaces touching, the only possible movement is rotational. It is impossible for the column to move backwards, forwards, sideways, upwards or downwards without the tins falling. Now try stacking the tins with a half-inch of spongy rubber between each one and you will find there is a full range of movement (see figure 1.4).

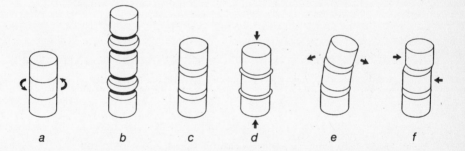

*Figure 1.4* The mechanical function of the discs. In diagram *a*, flat surface against flat surface allows only rotational movement; *b* and *c* show these surfaces with an added layer of elastic tissue (the intervertebral discs), permitting all kinds of movement; *d* shows compression, and *e* and *f* illustrate backwards, forwards, side to side and sliding motions.

Intervertebral discs give the spinal column freedom of movement, and provide it with a much greater ability to withstand blows than it would have without them.

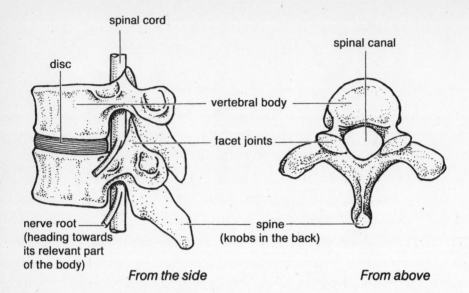

spinal cord

disc

spinal canal

vertebral body

facet joints

nerve root
(heading towards
its relevant part
of the body)

spine
(knobs in the back)

*From the side*

*From above*

*Figure 1.5* Vertebrae, facet joints, discs and nerves. See how the facet joints form to fit together, providing protection and support.

### Facet joints

With just vertebrae and intervertebral discs the spine would be flexible but floppy. You wouldn't want to entrust your body to such an unstable column, so nature has provided facet joints to stabilize the back and limit excessive movement. They also make it extremely difficult for vertebrae to become displaced.

Figure 1.5 illustrates how these joints are formed. An arch of bone projects from the back of each of the vertebral bodies. Four projections from each arch meet two corresponding ones from the arches above and two from the arches below to form slanting joints called facet joints.

The arches encase and protect the spinal cord. The spaces between the vertebrae and the arches are the neural canals through which the spinal nerves pass. As figure 1.5 shows, the floor of these neural canals is largely made up of the facet joints.

A nerve associated with each vertebra passes from the enclosed spinal cord through the canal formed by the arch and facet joint and on to the part of the body it supplies. This is the nerve root. Every nerve in the body comes from at least one root, and may come from several.

As we have already seen, the intervertebral discs allow a great deal of movement between the vertebrae, enabling them to squeeze together or to turn in a rotational movement. Obviously, it is important to keep this movement to a safe level and there are built-in restrictions in the form of muscles and ligaments as well as the facet joints. But it is the facet joints that bear the brunt of a blow or sharp jolt to the spine. Say, for example, you slip and sit down hard on the floor. The natural curve of the back increases, thus decreasing the effect of the blow. The discs will absorb much of the force by compressing. The facet joints, however, which have restricted movement, may be badly affected. The shock of the jolt could produce more movement than the facet joints are capable of accommodating and they may well be damaged.

Similarly, the type of jolt sustained in a car accident, or the twisting motion involved in a skiing accident may produce a range of attempted movement that the facet joints are not able to cope with and they are likely to be bruised.

Spinal muscles

Muscles are important to the spinal column. They have three main functions:

■ **Movement**. This is the most obvious one. Extremely intricate bundles of muscles run up and down the spinal column and control the movements of the spine in bending forward and backward, straightening up, bending from side to side and rotation. When you decide to perform a task such as walking or picking up an object, the motor centre of the brain is activated and sends a complex series of impulses to the various muscles involved.

■ **Maintenance of posture**. You may feel quite relaxed when you are sitting or standing still, but your muscles are actually working quite hard to stiffen and maintain the spinal curve so your body stays erect. If your spinal muscles were to be paralysed suddenly, say by the administration of a drug, your spine would promptly collapse and you would fall in a heap on the floor.

Static posture is usually maintained without any conscious effort on your part. Sensors determine the positions of the muscles, joints and ligaments and if the posture changes they react by sending impulses to the brain stem and the cerebellum, located at the base of the brain, which has overall control of posture. In response, appropriate impulses are sent out to instruct the muscles involved and restore the usual posture. Figure 1.6 shows the complex nature of the muscle layers in relation to the spine and the back.

---

SIT UP STRAIGHT!

It is a common belief that slouching is slovenly behaviour. However, since posture is controlled by the cerebellum, clearly this is not so. You can momentarily over-ride poor posture by exerting conscious control over the muscles and make an effort to sit or stand with a straight back, but as soon as you are distracted and stop thinking about it, the automatic mechanism takes over and the slouch returns.

Many people, especially children, are reprimanded for their poor posture when they can do little to correct it themselves. As discussed in chapter 3, a slouch is nearly always caused by back trouble. Once the underlying problem is treated there is a marked improvement in posture.

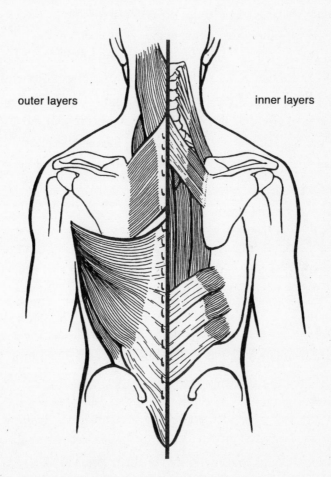

outer layers          inner layers

*Figure 1.6* The muscles in the back. Messages are sent to the brain stem and the cerebellum from each layer when any movement occurs, and posture is maintained.

■ **Muscle pump**. Muscles have a part to play in the circulation of the blood. Although this is probably the least known muscle function, it is crucial. You must appreciate this process if you are to gain a full understanding of the causes of back pain and related illnesses.

### Circulation of the blood

Blood is a complex fluid containing both red and white cells, as well as other substances including salts and antibodies. The red cells carry oxygen from the lungs around the body and then exchange it for carbon dioxide, which they return to the lungs. The white cells are scavengers and soldiers, engulfing foreign bodies, bacteria and viruses.

In a domestic central heating system, the central pump, under pressure, pushes water through the pipes to the radiators and then back to the pump where it is pumped out again. The heart resembles the central pump in that it pumps blood through the pipes – or arteries – to the tissues, but another force is needed to pump the blood back along the veins.

Blood leaves the heart through a large artery called the aorta and flows into smaller arteries, which branch off several times, becoming smaller each time. As their size decreases, the arteries' resistance to the flow progressively increases. The blood eventually passes through minute arterioles – by expanding and contracting, these control the exact quantity of blood received by the tissues – and into thin-walled vessels called capillaries. Figure 1.7 illustrates the movement of the blood from the heart through the body and back.

Most of the effort made by the heart is spent pushing the blood through the arterioles, so by the time it reaches the capillaries it exerts very little pressure. Having started at a pressure of 120 units, it reaches the beginning of the capillaries at 35 units. However, as the basic pressure in the tissue spaces between the capillaries is 15 units, the

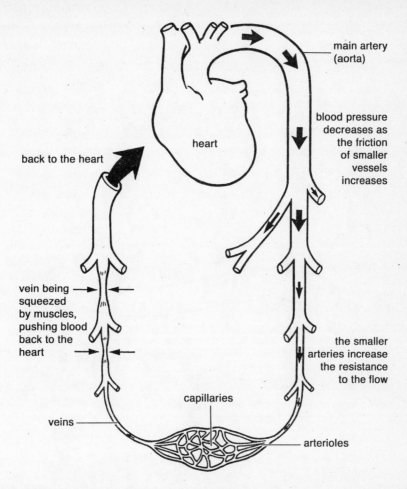

*Figure 1.7* The circulation of blood. As blood presure decreases, the muscles must work to return blood to the heart.

pressure is enough to force plasma – which is blood without the red cells – through the capillaries' thin walls and into the tissue spaces, where it becomes known as tissue fluid (see figure 1.8). This tissue fluid carries oxygen, which it exchanges for carbon dioxide and other waste products of tissue activity.

By the time the blood reaches just over halfway along a capillary, the pressure drops to around 10 or 15 units. Now the pressure in the tissue spaces is greater and this pushes the tissue fluid back into the capillary. When blood flows out of the capillaries into minute veins on its way back to the heart, its pressure is about 10 units. This is sufficient – along with the pumping effect of breathing and the constant rhythmic contractions of the vein walls, pushing blood ahead, like a piston – to maintain circulation when you are lying down or sleeping (see figure 1.9). However, as soon as you start to move about, extra pumping force is needed and this is where the muscle pump comes in.

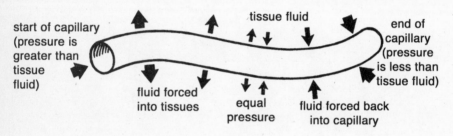

Figure 1.8 The circulation of fluid through a capillary. Higher pressure in the capillaries forces fluid out, and into the tissues. When the tissues reach a higher pressure, fluid is forced back into the capillary. The larger arrows indicate higher pressure.

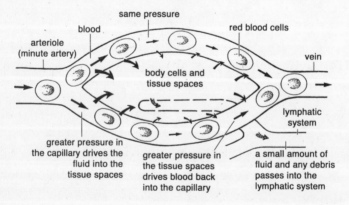

Figure 1.9 A larger view of capillary and tissue circulation.

## THE MUSCLE PUMP AT WORK

When a person is active, a large volume of blood needs to be returned to the heart. The greater the level of activity, the greater the amount of blood needed to nourish the hard-working muscles. Gravity helps to drain areas that are above the level of the heart, but the main mechanism for returning the blood from the tissues is the muscle pump.

When a muscle tightens – contracts, as it is called – it drives blood out of itself and into the veins. Non-return valves ensure that the flow is in one direction only – towards the heart. As the tightening muscles expand, they put pressure on the adjacent tissues, and this pressure drives tissue fluid back into the bloodstream and also compresses the veins so that the blood flows back to the heart more quickly (see figure 1.10a and b).

Later we will look at how back problems can interfere with the action of the muscle pump, leading to pain and also to many associated illnesses.

### Ligaments

Large bands of fibrous tissue, known as ligaments, run up and down the spinal column and wrap around the small joints (see figure 1.11), strengthening the spine, holding the bones together and generally acting in a supportive way. Ligaments could be described as doorstops, limiting excessive movement and preventing dislocation of both the large and small joints, and of the vertebrae.

Their composition is relatively primitive. Cells in tissues usually start life as simple structures, which become more and more complex as they become fully developed and able to perform the function of the particular tissue they make up. Fibrous tissue, however, has little

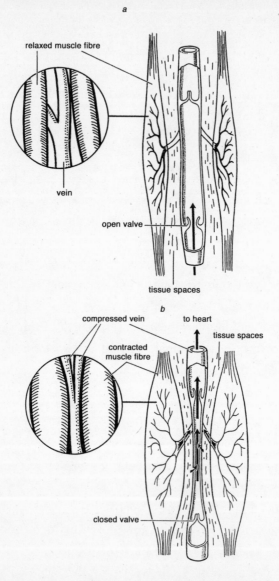

*a*

relaxed muscle fibre

vein

open valve

tissue spaces

*b*

compressed vein

to heart

contracted
muscle fibre

tissue spaces

closed valve

*Figure 1.10* The muscle pump. In diagram *a*, the relaxed muscle fibres allow veins and tissue spaces to fill with fluid. Diagram *b* indicates how contracting, bulging muscle fibres compress the tissue space and veins, squeezing the fluid into and up the veins. Valves ensure that the flow of blood goes only towards the heart.

ligaments

vertebral body

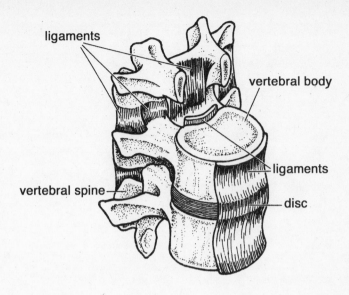

ligaments

vertebral spine

disc

*Figure 1.11* The ligaments of the spine are very strong, surrounding the discs and vertebrae to protect and support.

function other than support, so the cells remain simple. The ability to repair or reproduce is usually greatest in the simple cells and least in the most complex ones. So although ligaments can be torn in a severe injury, their powers of repair are quite considerable and they rarely sustain any lasting damage.

Sacro-iliac joints

These are large, flattish joints that fill the irregular gaps separating the sacrum (the fused lower part of the spinal column) from the iliac bones (the two bones that, fused together, form the complete pelvic basin). See figure 1.12. They are not moving joints, like the knee or shoulder. If they move at all, it is very, very little. They come into their own during pregnancy and childbirth when the powerful ligaments

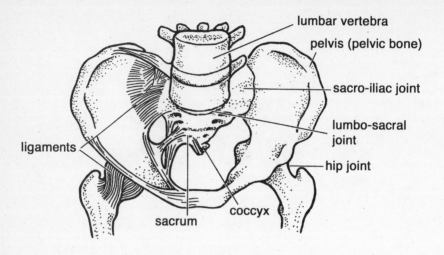

*Figure 1.12* The sacro-iliac joints, between the sacrum and the pelvis

attached to the joints soften to allow sufficient movement to open up
the pelvic gap.

## IN SUMMARY

The spine is made up of a number of bones placed one above the other.
These bones are separated by fibro-elastic discs, which are welded to
the vertebrae above and below. Arches projecting from the back of the
spinal column protect the spinal cord. The spaces between the arches
and each vertebral body form the neural canals through which the
spinal nerves pass.

The floor of these canals is largely made up of facet joints on either
side, which, with the discs, separate one vertebra from another. These
facet joints act like a natural corset to limit movement and stabilize the
back. The vertebrae form such strong and stable interlocking structures

that it is very difficult for them to be displaced unless the injury also fractures a bone.

Large muscles in the back maintain the posture of the spine and are responsible for performing and controlling movement.

Finally, ligaments run up and down the whole column and also surround the little joints, giving added stability and further helping to strengthen the spine.

## A SURPRISINGLY GOOD DESIGN

The spinal column is very well adapted for the job it has to do. Indeed, I find it hard to understand the common criticism that the back cannot cope with an upright life and is better suited to a primitive, four-legged existence. Would we suffer less back trouble if we were antelopes chasing around on all fours? Of course not. It is worth mentioning that animals also suffer from back problems. I have seen dogs and horses with backs as bad as any human's.

The common painful back is not a result of design faults but is caused by the stress we impose on it during everyday activities. The back performs its functions admirably, providing a firm but flexible base for the maintenance of our shape, the attachment of muscles and the protection of vital structures, especially the spinal cord. It is not, however, able to cope with the type of injury inflicted on it by modern life. Slipping and falling on to hard, man-made surfaces may well damage the spine, as will the falls and compressional injuries that are part and parcel of games such as rugby football. The somewhat more spectacular damage incurred in a skiing accident or falling downstairs, and the altogether different injuries resulting from falling from a horse or being involved in a car accident are more examples.

Most of us take little exercise to keep the circulation going, and spend a lot of time sitting down, neither of which help the back. Business, domestic and financial worries, as we shall see later, also place an unnatural strain on our resources. We eat foods that may disagree with our system. Certain foods such as milk and other dairy products, or white flour and additives, can cause a reaction in some people that increases any inflammation in the body, wherever it may be present, and this considerably aggravates back trouble. In the West we tend to over-eat, which puts yet another load on our skeletal system.

Despite all this, the body is usually able to cope – as long as it remains uninjured. The back is so beautifully formed that I believe it is impossible to blame the mechanics of the spinal column for back pain. In the following chapters we will look at the real causes of back problems.

# 2 YOUR PAINFUL BACK

## The cause of recurrent chronic back pain

Experts tend to agree on the causes and management of well-recognized, diagnosable diseases of the spine, such as tumours, ankylosing spondylitis (where the vertebrae gradually become stiff, fixed and painful with associated arthritis of the hips), Paget's disease (thickening of the bones), fractures and spondylolisthesis (where one vertebra slips forward on another). However, the majority of those troubled by back pain do not suffer from any of these specific illnesses and they are grouped together as having non-specific back pain. For patients who have nothing very definite to explain their back pain, the answers are as varied as they are vague.

## CONFUSION AND CONTROVERSY

There must be more controversy about the cause of recurring non-specific back pain than about almost any other subject in medicine. The saying that if you go to 10 different consultants you will get 10 different opinions is probably true. The medical profession is likely to suggest a number of reasons for non-specific back pain, including protruding or ruptured discs, wear, strained muscles or ligaments, a strained or displaced sacro-iliac joint and bad posture. Many doctors believe that back pain has psychological causes (see chapter 3).

Alternative practitioners have their own theories, depending on their particular discipline. Osteopaths and chiropractors will blame displaced or misaligned vertebrae, displaced discs and back strain. Relaxation therapists blame the patient's posture.

Some say the pain is a result of carrying heavy weights or lifting objects in an ill-advised way. Others believe diet is at the root of the problem, or blame worry and mental stress.

Now I am about to add my own theory – without, I hope, adding to the confusion – to explain how pain comes about and why it is intermittent, and to show that the underlying cause has a number of other effects on the body.

## THAT OLD INJURY

Virtually every patient I have seen with chronic or recurring back pain has at some time in the past suffered an injury that involved a sharp jolt, jerk or twist. It is my belief that these injuries are the cause of back problems. Many of my patients find this difficult to understand at first. Indeed, sometimes the initial injury occurred so long ago that they need a lot of prompting to recall what happened.

Jim, 37, had been complaining of pain in the lumbar region on and off for about seven years. He had no idea what had brought it on. When the pain first started it was an inconveniencing ache. After a while, however, it became more frequent and more severe. Over the years, he noticed that his back was often uncomfortable when getting up, either from bed or after sitting for any period of time, and after prolonged standing. Driving a car had become difficult as he felt a sharp pain after about half an hour.

After examining him, I felt reasonably sure that the back trouble was caused by an old injury. Jim couldn't remember any such injury but his wife recalled an incident about 12 years before when he'd fallen down 10 stairs. Jim had undergone treatment for the original bruising but had put the episode completely out of his mind.

How could I be so confident that Jim's past injury was the cause of his intermittent back pain? After all, he had been free of pain for five years before he felt any symptoms.

### Five forms of illness

First of all, we need to look at the five different basic forms of illness in humans – congenital problems, infections, tumours and growths, degenerative conditions and injuries – and consider them in relation to painful back syndrome. By a process of elimination we can see why injury is almost always the culprit.

- **Congenital problems**, such as an extra or split vertebra, are malformations present at birth. They are usually fairly easy to diagnose and are likely to cause trouble, *if at all*, from an early age. There is little chance of them starting to cause symptoms later in life, which is when most back trouble begins. Most congenital problems show in an X-ray. In general, they are unlikely to be involved in the type of back pain we are looking at here.

- **Infections** are caused by bacteria, or occasionally a virus, and have definite signs and symptoms – the affected area becomes hot and pulsates; there is swelling, pain and loss of function. Infections will often show up on an X-ray, and cause the patient to feel unwell and possibly to have an abnormal temperature. They may alter the blood count and thus be shown up by a blood test.

Infections usually come on rapidly and are either quickly cleared as the body's defences overcome them, or can be treated with an appropriate drug. Longer-lasting ones can be readily diagnosed. Very rarely, infections can be surgically removed.

So it is not difficult to recognize infections. They are relatively sudden in onset, unlikely to linger for years and have a predictable end. Infections can usually be eliminated as a cause of chronic or recurring back pain.

■ **Tumours and growths** are also fairly easy to diagnose. Once the pain has started, there are seldom remissions, especially after a few weeks, and intensity increases steadily as time goes on. Growths in the spine are often secondary to a tumour elsewhere and are usually diagnosed in the initial stages – long before the back pain starts. Persistent intermittent back trouble over many years is almost never due to tumours or growths so these can also be eliminated as possible causes.

■ **Degenerative conditions** are often blamed for causing back-pain syndrome. People are led to believe that back pain is just another part of getting old. *I am adamant that this is not so.* Ageing and degeneration are quite different processes. Just because you are advancing in years does not mean you, or your back, are wearing out. When patients of 60 plus are successfully treated they remain free of pain for many years.

DEGENERATION IS NOT THE CULPRIT

Ageing is so often blamed for non-specific back pain that it is important to take a closer look at it and to define the difference between ageing and degeneration.

**Ageing** is a physiological change where tissues become less efficient and virile. This process is designed to end in death. It is nature's way of making continuous replacement possible and so allowing for natural selection to continue improving the species as time goes by. As a slowing down of the repair mechanism takes place with age so actual performance lessens. The level of wear and tear is always matched by the ability to repair.

**Degeneration** occurs under extreme circumstances only, when tissues are subjected to protracted excessive strain or when the repair mechanism becomes defective and the tissues involved cannot keep pace with normal wear and tear. The body may attempt to repair the area but the efforts are usually fruitless as nothing can be done to stop degeneration under these circumstances. Under normal conditions, tissues do not degenerate. There is no reason to suppose that the back is any different from the rest of the body.

**X-rays** show up abnormalities in the back, especially an increase in the density and size of bone at joint margins. I believe this is usually due to a compensatory strengthening reaction to the considerable pressure put on the spine by the protective spasms of the muscles as a result of an injury sustained possibly years before. *It is regeneration, not degeneration*. A spasm is a contraction of the muscles caused by the bruising of the facet joints, and is intended to stiffen the back to give these joints a rest and a chance to recover. It has nothing to do with degeneration.

Bone is living tissue that is permanently readjusting and adapting to any change in need or circumstance. A porter constantly carrying heavy loads would develop stronger and denser bones in his legs than he had before. Similarly, if the pressure of a muscle spasm is putting great strain on a joint surface, the joint can be expected to enlarge to meet the challenge. Unfortunately, the extra bone around the edge of a joint is not well formed and is usually irregular in shape.

Another change often apparent in X-rays is a narrowing of the spaces between the vertebrae. Again, this is not usually caused by degeneration of the discs but by the pressure from the protective spasm, which compresses them.

As both these changes are a normal reaction to the pressure brought about by a spasm, they would not in themselves cause pain. This is borne out by the fact that the degree or extent of changes in X-ray pictures bears almost no relationship to the amount or severity of pain. On a number of occasions, X-rays taken of organs such as the kidneys have also shown very advanced changes in the spine, yet the patients deny back pain. Similarly, a number of the very worst back-pain sufferers I have seen have had completely normal X-rays.

These are some of the reasons why I do not accept that degeneration is the usual cause of back-pain syndrome.

■ **Injury** is, in almost all cases, found to be the cause of recurrent, chronic back pain, the other groups having been eliminated. In many cases, such as Jim's, there is a long quiescent period after the immediate effects of the original injury have settled before the patient first suffers pain. Often, a second and sometimes quite minor injury will set it off.

Susan, 43, was strong, athletic and keen on sports. When she came to see me a year ago she was in so much pain she could hardly move, and very perplexed about the cause of it. She said she had never had any real trouble with her back, although she did feel a little stiff after long car journeys. The attack came suddenly, quite out of the blue.

Her story is a common one. She had returned from a holiday abroad, the journey involving a considerable amount of sedentary travelling and carrying of heavy cases. When she arrived home she went into the kitchen to make a cup of tea, leaned forward to lift a cup from the shelf and was seized by agonizing pain in the lumbar region. The pain didn't respond to bed rest, painkillers or anti-inflammatory drugs.

After four days, she was brought, with some difficulty, to see me. She was under the impression that reaching for the cup was the cause of the pain but could not understand why. Examination was difficult as movement was so painful, but I could see the muscle spasm and that the normal lumbar curve of her back was flattened. This gave me enough evidence to suspect that the real trouble was not due to the stretching action but to an injury sustained some years previously when she had probably slipped and sat down hard. Reaching for the cup had merely been the precipitating factor in the onset of pain.

Susan remembered an accident on a skiing holiday six years previously when she had slipped on the ice outside her hotel in Switzerland and fallen on her bottom. She was a little shaken up at the time but had soon recovered and was able to carry on skiing without any problems. Indeed, she felt pleased that she had done herself no serious damage. Once the initial discomfort had passed, there were no symptoms and she had put the incident to the back of her mind.

It was only when Susan felt the sudden cramp in her back muscles that she was aware she had trouble. The previous jolt had caused a wave of pressure up her spine, compressing the discs and thus jolting the facet joints and bruising them (see figure 2.1). Although there had been no symptoms for several years, the underlying problem remained and the stretching action of reaching for the cup had sparked off the pain. So how is it that a minor incident can precipitate an agonizing attack?

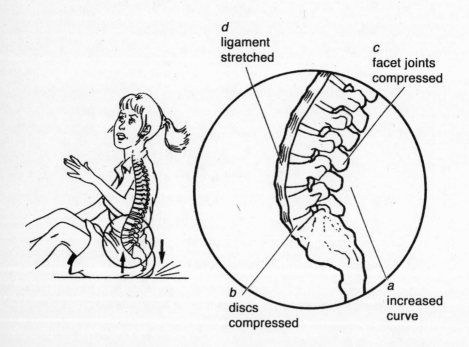

*Figure 2.1* The effect of a blow to the spine. At point *a*, the spine has increased its curve to absorb the shock; *b* shows the compression of the discs (greatest at the lower end); *c* indicates how the blow affects the facet joints, which limit movement, and *d* illustrates the stretched ligament.

## The last straw

It is understandable that Susan should put the blame for the pain on stretching for the cup. This was, after all, her first experience of acute back pain. Similarly, many sufferers believe that their pain is due to straining their backs by lifting or trying to lift a heavy weight – usually a heavy suitcase or piece of furniture. A common tale is that they were trying to push a car when suddenly there was a 'click' in the back and they were immediately in agony.

I doubt that a voluntary effort such as lifting or straining could cause a back injury. If you are straining unsuccessfully to unscrew a jam-jar top, do you worry that you might damage the muscles in your forearm and hand? Of course not. You can either undo it or you can't. You don't expect to be laid up in bed for days with a painful forearm simply because you tried. So why should you expect dramatic problems if you push any other part of the body to the limit of muscular effort? It seems strange that it should be so universally agreed that the back alone will suffer under these circumstances. As we have already seen, the back is particularly well adapted to the work it has to do.

The impossibility of this commonly held belief is borne out by looking at the physiology of the skeletal system. Our muscles, tendons, ligaments and joints all have a large number of sensors, which measure and monitor every function of every tissue. There are many different types of sensor, each one with a particular function, such as measuring blood pressure, body temperature, the degree of bend in a joint or skin sensations. One type detects the pulling strain on the tissue. These sensors work to protect the area from self-inflicted damage and are called Golgi tendon organs. Once a certain level of strain has been reached, which is considerably below that which could damage the tissue, the organs react by sending out impulses to counteract those going to the muscles. This restricts the muscular effort if the pull becomes too great. Excess effort is therefore limited before it reaches a level when harm could be caused.

In almost every patient, like Susan, who pinpoints a minor injury such as straining or lifting as the start of back pain, there is a history of a much more serious incident some years before. This previous injury will have produced far greater stresses in the back than could be reached by voluntary effort and, I believe, is the real cause of the back problem. The trouble is latent for a period of time, surfacing only when pain is triggered by a much less traumatic activity.

## A SHOCK TO THE SYSTEM

If an old injury is the cause of back problems, we must now examine the possible effects of that injury. What does it do to the back? Why does it cause intermittent pain? Why does the pain vary so much in its severity? Why is there so often a long, symptomless period before a sudden attack of pain? What is the progress of events? To explain, let us consider the example of someone who falls a short distance and sits down very heavily on a hard floor. Figure 2.1 illustrates damage done by this kind of injury. Patricia had had just such an accident.

Patricia came to see me when she was 32. She said she had suffered back trouble on and off since she was in her teens. In the last two or three years it had been ruining her life. Whatever she did was painful. Unlike so many patients, she could vividly recall the initial injury that sparked the problem. She was 15 and enjoying a disco with a new boyfriend. After a particularly energetic dance, he suggested they have a drink.

Now this practical joker thought he'd try a trick on Patricia. He pulled up a chair for her but just as she was about to sit down he yanked it away. She went crashing on to the dance floor, giving her back a very nasty bump. Needless to say she didn't think it was at all funny. The boyfriend didn't last long, but the problem lingered on.

An injury such as Susan's or Patricia's results in:

- increased flexion of the normal curves of the back, particularly the lumbar curve, which is the first to be affected by the blow
- a compressional force directly through the vertebrae and discs
- a hard jolt to the lumbo-sacral joint at the base of the spine and the sacro-iliac joints between the spine and the pelvis
- sharp stretching of the ligament and possibly the muscles, both of which may be torn
- bruising of the facet joints, the primary functions of which are to stabilize the vertebrae and to limit movement in nearly all directions.

When nature doesn't know best

Nature responds to the bruising of any joint in the body by trying to protect it and help it repair itself. The emergency repair mechanism, seen as an inflammatory reaction, ensures that the blood supply is greatly increased to the affected tissues, thus bringing extra oxygen and nutrients. In addition, the sensors in the joint, which are specially designed to detect bruising and inflammation, will send impulses along the nerve to the spinal cord where they cross directly to the motor nerves and via them to the muscles which move the joint. The impulses put the muscles into a protective contraction called a spasm. The number of impulses coming from the bruised joint controls the level of the spasm – the more severe the bruising, the stronger the contraction.

PROTECTIVE SPASM

The spasm is a perfectly normal contraction of the muscle, controlled by the nerves. It is the body's way of promoting repair of the bruising and we are completely unaware of it occurring. The idea is that the spasm acts as a kind of splint or corset. By stiffening the joint to prevent or limit movement, the joint surfaces should be given a recuperative rest.

Unlike an agonizing muscle cramp, there are no symptoms when a muscle is in spasm. While a spasm is a controlled normal contraction sent down the usual nerve route, a cramp is uncontrolled, originating in the muscle itself through some internal fault. The intensity of the pull in a bad cramp is sufficient to produce a pain that has been described as an oversized spear stuck in the area.

In many instances, the protective spasm works well. Unfortunately, in the case of the back, nature doesn't get it right. Putting the muscles across the facet joint into a protective spasm produces exactly the opposite effect to the one intended. It actually maintains the injury to the joint instead of enabling it to heal quickly. Why? Let's look at what goes wrong with nature's healing powers.

As we have seen in chapter 1, the facet joints are small and relatively inflexible. By comparison, the muscles in the spine are large and powerful. Given this, the pressure of the muscle spasm on the facet joints is obviously tremendous. In fact, the pressure has been measured

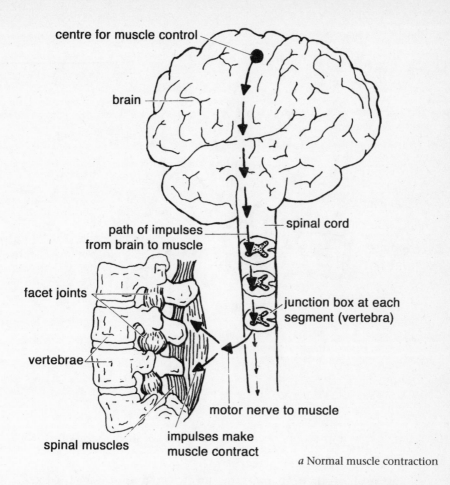

centre for muscle control

brain

path of impulses
from brain to muscle

spinal cord

facet joints

junction box at each
segment (vertebra)

vertebrae

motor nerve to muscle

spinal muscles

impulses make
muscle contract

*a* Normal muscle contraction

*Figure 2.2* In diagram *a*, a voluntary muscle contraction, the movement is started in the brain, travelling down the spinal cord, arriving at the junction box at the correct level in the spinal cord, and passing from the junction box to the muscle, causing it to contract. In diagram *b*, a muscle spasm, the impulses start in a bruised facet joint, and they pass to the junction box, via the same nerve, causing an identical contraction.

at up to 30lb per square inch. However, due to the mechanics of the spine, the spasm does little to limit movement. Think of it this way – could you limit the already small movement of two tins joined

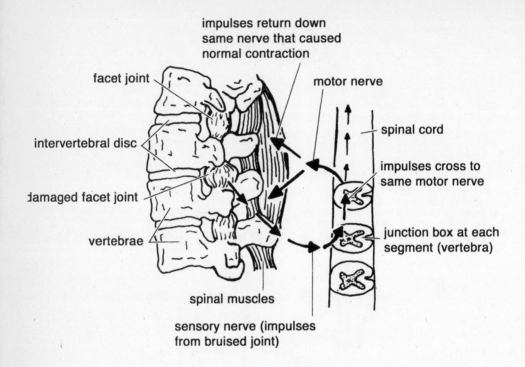

impulses return down
same nerve that caused
normal contraction

motor nerve

facet joint

spinal cord

intervertebral disc

impulses cross to
same motor nerve

damaged facet joint

vertebrae

junction box at each
segment (vertebra)

spinal muscles

sensory nerve (impulses
from bruised joint)

*b* Contraction of a muscle spasm

together by a soft rubber pad by tying a piece of string tightly on either side?

So we have the unhappy situation where a joint, which can still move fairly freely, is subjected to considerable extra pressure as well as the normal stresses and strains of ordinary life.

### Why are there no symptoms?

With so much happening, it may seem surprising that there is no pain. In fact, any mild sensations of pain arising from the bruising of the facet joints are suppressed by the brain so that you are no longer aware of them. Put simply, the brain doesn't want to know about it if it can't do anything to change the situation. It's rather like being in a room with a bad smell or continuous noise. After a while, you gradually get so used to it that you do not notice it at all.

With no obvious symptoms over a long period of time, most people believe their backs have made a full recovery. Indeed, as I was going through a batch of several hundred case histories recently, I found that there was an average of 11 years from an original injury to the first symptoms becoming noticeable.

Although no pain is experienced during this time, other signs may indicate trouble with the spine. One is that the protective spasm of the muscles makes them feel very firm; another is that the pull of the muscles often alters the normal curve of the back. Try contracting the muscles of your arm – feel the firmness. That is what I am looking for when I examine a patient by palpation (diagnosis by touch). To show just how evident a spasm is on touch, consider the story of a skiing friend of mine.

Leo phoned me a few years ago to say that his back was troubling him a great deal. On examination I diagnosed his trouble as being due to an old injury, mainly because I could feel the firm protective spasm of the back muscles. After several sessions of treatment he was pain-free and the spasm had almost completely gone.

Two years later, Leo and his wife invited me to a dinner party during which he complained that his back was as bad as it had been before he came to see me. Being rather surprised by this, I asked to have a quick look at it and we retired to another room. When I felt his back, I found there was a great deal of recent bruising but very little evidence of the firm protective spasm I had originally treated. I explained that this was not the original problem but a fairly recent injury to his back.

Leo denied that he had injured his back recently, but while I was still brooding over the problem, our hostess proudly switched on a video of her husband skiing. It was quite a revelation. One moment Leo was coming down the mountain at 60 miles per hour, the next he had disappeared in a cloud of snow and when it had settled, there was no sign of Leo or his skis. It was lucky, he said, that they were taking the video or he wouldn't have been found so quickly. He had fallen down an eight-foot-deep hole and had been knocked out with all the snow on top of him. And this was the man who said he had not injured his back since I had last treated him!

Dorothy, a 38-year-old mother, came to see me five years ago. She had fallen downstairs 20 years before and had hurt herself but felt fortunate there was no serious injury. She had noticed that her back ached after long car journeys or sitting for any length of time but as this went away so quickly, she did not worry about it. Then, seven years ago, while she was bathing her child, she leant over and her back went 'click'. It was agony at the time and had remained troublesome.

Dorothy tried osteopathy, physiotherapy, acupuncture and drugs. Some were helpful but just for a short time. She complained of bad pain in the lumbar region and occasionally it was so severe it radiated down the leg.

As I examined her back, I could feel the distinct spasm of the paravertebral muscles (the ones that run up and down the back between the vertebrae) from the lower half of the thoracic spine to the low lumbar region, particularly in the mid-lumbar region. She had seven visits by which time the spasm had largely gone, and she has been free of back trouble ever since.

Let's look at what happened to Dorothy's back when she fell downstairs all those years ago. Her spine received a blow and bruising to the facet joints, and nature tried to protect the joint and promote healing in its usual way by putting the muscles into spasm. However, the pressure on these joints was so strong that it maintained the injury. For many years Dorothy was unaware that she had any problem. Then the bathtime incident sparked off the pain by stretching and overworking the muscles, causing them to go into a painful cramp.

---

**See you in court**

This delay in the appearance of the symptoms can give rise to problems in obtaining compensation for injuries sustained at work, for example, or in a car accident. I have been called upon to give evidence in court cases where there is some dispute about the reason for the current pain and the disruption it causes to everyday activities. I have had to satisfy the court that it really was the injury that occurred many years before that was at the root of the problem.

---

LEADING UP TO AN ATTACK

The next question we must ask is why, after such a long, trouble-free period, patients have an attack of pain followed by intermittent attacks. To answer this, we need to study the sequence of events that leads from the silent stage to the attack of pain. I hope the diagrams will help clarify my explanation of this rather complex process. You may also like to refer back to the previous chapter.

As we have seen, one of the functions of the muscles is the part they play in the circulation of the blood. The blood's pressure is determined by the expansion and contraction of the arterioles through which it flows on its way into the capillaries. Where plasma is diffused from the capillaries into the tissues, blood is at low pressure.

To continue the analogy of the domestic central heating system used earlier, imagine radiators made of thin latex rubber. The water would flow into them, expanding them, and have no force left to go on. The radiators would need to be squeezed to push the water out and into the pipes leading back to the pump, and relaxed to enable them to refill ready to be squeezed again.

In the body, the muscles administer the squeeze and so provide the force required to pump the blood onward. Every time a muscle contracts it tightens and squeezes out blood into tiny veins. The blood flows on into bigger and bigger veins and non-return valves make this a one-way traffic system back to the heart. The contracted muscle also squeezes the adjacent tissues thus spreading the pumping effect (see figure 2.3a and b).

*When a muscle is in spasm following an injury, its alternate relaxation and contraction is interfered with.* The spasm increases the supply of blood to the muscle to help it cope with the extra work caused by the permanent contraction, but reduces the efficiency of the muscle pump. Fluid diffuses out of the blood and builds up in the tissue spaces, where it is called oedema (see figure 2.4a and b). This waterlogging, which creates a situation rather like a traffic jam, means that there is a less effective blood supply in precisely the area where most blood is required for the body's repair mechanism to work. An extra-large supply is needed to speed up the healing process and also to carry extra supplies to overworked contracting muscles.

### Building up to a critical level

The symptoms of back injury may not show for several years because, together with the other forces that return blood to the heart – gravity

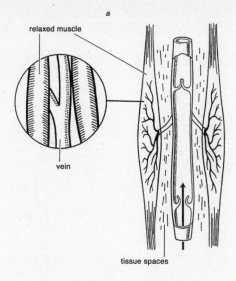

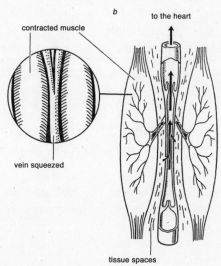

*Figure 2.3* In diagram *a*, the thin, relaxed muscle exerts little pressure, allowing the veins and tissue spaces to fill. In diagram *b*, however, you can see how the hard, contracting muscle exerts pressure. It squeezes the blood back to the heart, the valves ensuring one-way flow.

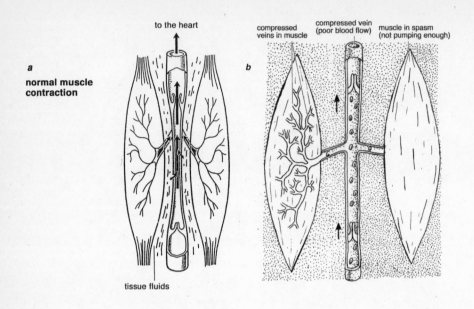

Figure 2.4 Diagram *a* illustrates a normal contraction, which allows fluid to circulate by squeezing the veins and tissue spaces. In diagram *b*, the muscle in spasm is permanently contracted, and this does not allow the veins to refill – or to be squeezed out again. The pumping action becomes slower and slower as the tissue fluids clog and collect in the tissue spaces.

and the residual pressure in the veins – there may be just enough movement of the back to keep things reasonably in order. In this case, the build-up of oedema does not cause a major upset. However, during all this time the muscles and adjacent tissues are suffering from the cumulative effects of the gradual increase in waste products and lack of oxygen.

It's not surprising that under those conditions there is a delay in healing, or even deterioration in the condition of the affected facet joints. Over the years, as the joints further deteriorate, the protective spasm increases and is followed by a worsening of the traffic jam. As a muscle spasm is a normal contraction, the patient feels no pain, but eventually the situation reaches the stage when the muscle can no longer function normally and goes into a cramp. As explained, this is an abnormal contraction generated in the muscle itself and this is what produces pain. If only a few of the thousand muscle fibres are affected, the patient will feel a slight ache. If more fibres are affected, the pain is proportionally greater. If the whole muscle is in cramp, the pain is agonizing.

## THE ONSET OF PAIN

The six common precipitating factors of pain are as follows:

- **Muscular effort**. This can be quick and intense, such as lifting a heavy weight, or less arduous but more prolonged, such as digging the garden. Both cause more blood than usual to circulate to the working muscles to supply the extra oxygen required and remove the waste products. There is a critical point for the muscles in spasm when not enough oxygen is getting through and, due to that and the build-up of waste products, the muscles go into cramp.

- **Complete rest**. If the muscle is already in spasm, rest will further reduce the effect of the muscle pump to an inadequate level and there comes a point, as above, when a cramp will ensue.

- **Viral infection.** A number of common viruses invade the whole body and any susceptible tissues will be attacked. They often choose the muscles of the back and joints, so any virus infection, such as the common cold, can be the cause of a sudden bout of acute back pain. The diagnosis is often missed, partly because an infection is not considered and also because the patient has often done something, such as lifting a case, that automatically takes the blame. The diagnosis can often be confirmed by some other manifestation of an infection, such as feeling unusually tired or displaying the obvious signs of a mild cold or sore throat, however slight, or having aches in some other joints, such as the hips, knees or hands. The infection can cause a single attack of pain, but is not, of course, a cause of ongoing chronic back problems.

■ **Tonsils.** Although tonsillitis is an infection, the tonsils are such an important cause of back trouble as a whole, and the commonest single cause of a chronic back problem that refuses to clear up, that they deserve a separate entry.

We are designed by nature to eat infected foods, so the throat has to have powerful safeguards against infection becoming out of control. Tonsils are like a factory directly in the throat that takes bacteria into 'test tubes', cultures them and produces antibodies against that particular bug. Any future attack of that infection, especially if the throat has been scratched by a bone, is already nine-tenths dealt with by the already present antibodies. By the time children are about six years old, they will have come into contact with just about all the ordinary bugs they are likely to meet, and the tonsils gradually stop functioning.

Unfortunately, owing to the fact that life is now so different from the primitive one for which we were designed, we may meet a virulent bacterium, such as a haemolytic streptococcus, that breaks through the test tube and invades and destroys the tonsils them-selves. This is like having dead-end kids invading a munitions factory and causing an explosion that wrecks it, leaving the kids in possession. Apart from mugging passers-by causing sore throats and colds, they discover that the water supply to the town (the body) lies underneath the factory and inject poisons into it. Thus the water causes trouble down in the town. In the body, these toxins inflame the linings of joints, especially ones that are already damaged, such as those involved in back trouble.

If a person has sore throats, or has had them in the past, the tonsils need examining and almost certainly removing. Throat specialists may advise leaving the tonsils in if the infection does not seem too bad but, in my opinion, it is important that infected tonsils are removed as, apart from the back, they can make you feel unwell and unusually tired. (My book *Get Well, Stay Well* has more information on this subject, and see also Appendix 5, page 277.)

■ **Posture.** An increased curve of the spine alters the shape of the muscles, stretching some groups and making them much more likely to go into a painful cramp than would be the case with normal, unstretched muscles.

■ **Stretching the muscle**. A bending or twisting movement often sets off pain. The stretching raises the pressure in the muscle, which already has excess fluid in it, and this causes its monitoring sensors to send out impulses that lead to violent correcting contractions, trying to oppose the stretching and restore the muscle to its normal length. This has the same effect as quick and intense muscular effort and can cause an immediate cramp. Stretching under slow, controlled conditions, however, can be beneficial to people with back trouble because it activates the muscle pump.

REACHING CRISIS POINT

The final question we must address in this chapter is why there can be such a difference in the severity of the incident that sets off the pain.

Why does one person suffer an attack of pain doing something as seemingly effortless as bending to tie a shoelace while someone else reaches crisis level only when single-handedly reorganizing the furniture in the lounge?

Much depends on the condition of the muscle. If it is extremely close to the critical point with the build-up of waste products and lack of oxygen, just a small effort, such as leaning forward slightly to look in a mirror, is all that is necessary to produce the cramp. If the muscle is not yet near crisis point with moderate oxygen reserves and not too excessive a build-up of waste, it might take a very big muscular effort, such as trying to push a car, to put the muscle into a sudden cramp. The tremendous increase in oxygen requirements and build-up of waste products may be enough to bridge the gap.

# 3 YOUR BACK IN QUESTION

## Clear answers to common queries

This chapter uses my theory of the cause of non-specific back pain to offer logical explanations to questions that puzzle so many people.

*Why is my back so often at its worst first thing in the morning?*

It seems strange to many people that their backs should be troublesome when they've been in bed for some time. This is the very time you would expect it to be well rested, and after all, doctors often advise bed rest for bad backs. However, rest actually aggravates the underlying problem.

As we have seen in the previous chapter, when a muscle is in spasm there is an increased supply of blood to the muscles and tissues, but the muscle pump does not work efficiently. Extra tissue fluid, or oedema, builds up, leading to an increase in waste products and oxygen deficiency. When you are asleep your muscle pump is at an all-time low. Oedema accumulates until it reaches a maximum level which, from the experiences of my patients, seems to be around three in the morning or later. The pain often wakes them. The worst moment is often experienced when the sufferer tries to get out of bed. By this time even slight muscular effort is enough to cause a cramp.

When you get up and move around some of the fluid is squeezed out of the tissue spaces, improving the circulation, and the likelihood of a painful cramp diminishes. In a short time, the back can become symptom-free and comfortable.

*Why is it that I can manage a fairly energetic task such as digging in the garden and not feel any pain, only to be in agony once I sit down?*

This curious fact makes sense when you think about it. While you are gardening, the movement of the back muscles is sufficient to squeeze out enough blood to keep them below the threshold of pain, despite the increased blood supply to the muscles brought about by the effort. However, this increased blood supply does not immediately diminish when the digging stops. It continues for some hours after the work is finished and, because the pumping effect is greatly reduced when the body is at rest, causes a steady increase in tissue fluid and floods the muscles out. So later in the day, or even the next day, you experience pain when you are simply watching television or relaxing in bed.

*Why does exercise help?*

Patients often extol the benefits of exercise. A daily swim or gentle workout is the ticket to a pain-free life. The trouble is that once regular exercise ceases, the intermittent pain starts again.

Charles was 20 when he was involved in a car accident. He suffered a mild whiplash injury but the symptoms disappeared very rapidly, without any treatment. He was badly shaken up at the time. Ten years later, he felt a click in his back as he picked up his three-year-old daughter. He sought help from an osteopath, who relieved him of the pain, but from then on Charles started to complain of painful twinges in his back when he got up in the morning and after long journeys.

On the advice of a friend, Charles took up yoga. He was overjoyed at how much it helped ease the aches and pains. He kept it up for nearly three years and was relatively symptom-free during this time. Then he got a job promotion, which meant a busy schedule and no time for yoga. Only a month after stopping the regular activity he started to experience pain in his back again.

Exercise may relieve the pain but it often does little to correct the basic problem. It works by activating the muscle pump and so decreasing the likelihood of the muscle going into a cramp. The muscles are prevented from turning a constant protective spasm into a cramp by regular exercise. Once the exercise stops, it does not take long for the muscles to move into a critical state. People often mistakenly believe that it is the building up of muscles that makes the back feel better.

*Does age affect back problems?*

I am often asked whether age makes any difference to the severity of back trouble. 'Can you help my mother? She is nearly eighty and has been told she is now too old for treatment to work', is one example. In my experience, people of a mature age respond to treatment more quickly and easily than most other age groups. By the time a person reaches the age of 65 his or her muscles begin to weaken and probably take on less stress. It follows that the spasm could also be weaker. In many cases, the back undergoes a spontaneous improvement around this time.

Gladys, aged 73, came to see me because she had a painful right knee. She had damaged it about six months previously. It had not recovered and was actually slowly deteriorating. It was the only joint in her body to be affected so I asked her, among other things, whether she had had back trouble. She said that she had suffered back pain on and off for many years but that in the last five years she'd had much less pain and had more or less forgotten about it. The telltale spasm could be felt, and after it had been treated, her knee made a slow but good recovery.

Young people often seem to be able to cope with an injury without suffering any pain for many years. This is probably because they have a resilient repair mechanisms and usually move about a great deal, even though the muscles are in spasm. When they reach their twenties or thirties and are less actively engaged, their repair mechanisms stop doing such a good job. The traffic-jam situation in the back begins to worsen and the person may well start suffering episodes of pain. *It is also possible that the childhood aches and pains that adults so readily label growing pains are actually the start of back trouble.*

*Will I get better quicker if I am very fit?*

No. The level of fitness and general muscle strength of the sufferer has a profound effect on the course of the treatment, but in exactly the opposite way to what you'd expect. In an extremely fit person, spasm is tremendous. These people may experience pain more easily and the pain may be more severe. Many tough men have been brought to tears by it.

One of the most worrying patients that I have ever treated was a man who had recently been the world's non-Japanese judo champion. He was about 5ft 8ins tall and seemed about the same width. The muscles in his back were absolutely enormous and felt as big as an average person's thigh. He had suffered back trouble for some years and had attacks of extremely severe pain.

I was almost worn out every time I treated him because the spasm in his back produced a resistance that must have been two or three times more than an average person's. When I got him, say, 75 per cent better, the spasm or pressure of the back muscles on the joints was still probably as great as that of a less fit person at their worst. The number of treatments that he needed for a full recovery was three or four times more than usual.

*Why is my back so painful after a long journey?*

You may well find that two of the worst things for your back trouble are sitting for long periods in a chair and, even more worrying, in a car or aeroplane. Indeed, a car journey is probably about the most difficult situation that an injured back can be asked to tolerate.

Let's consider what happens to your back when you are immobilized in the sitting position. The back muscles are stretched as the thighs extend at a right angle. A poorly supported back will become more curved, which will stretch the muscles. In addition, the limited movement diminishes the muscle pump.

Now add the motion of the car. The muscles in your back will have to work hard consistently to keep you upright against the stresses of a motorcar in action. When turning corners, the muscles have to resist the trunk lurching sideways; when braking, they must resist the body falling forwards; and when accelerating, they may have to resist some backward movement.

There will also be little jolts through the spine from bumps on the road, which may increase the bruising of the facet joints fractionally, and thus the spasm of the back.

It's hardly surprising that a car journey should give rise to problems. However, once the journey is over and you start to move about, the muscle pump is restored and the trouble soon subsides. For this reason, it is wise to plan a series of short stops on a long journey. Keep the muscle pump activated by taking a little exercise – even walking around the car can be enough.

*Is bad posture the cause of back pain?*

Many of us can recall countless childhood reprimands for poor posture. If you have children, you probably make a point of correcting them for slouching and stooping. However, as we saw in chapter 1, we have very little voluntary control over our posture. In general, posture is controlled by an automatic mechanism based in the cerebellum, which controls repetitive functions in the body. If, say, the body tilts forwards a little in an involuntary movement, muscles tightening to pull the body back into a normal posture will automatically correct this. If, however, the back is injured and some groups of muscles have gone into spasm and thus an increased contraction, it is easy to see that normal posture can be upset. The curve of the back would either be increased much as the tightening strings on a bow, or, if the opposite group of muscles is affected, the normal curve would tend to be flattened (see figure 3.1).

Many people believe poor posture leads to back pain, but slouching and stooping are the effect of back trouble rather than the cause.

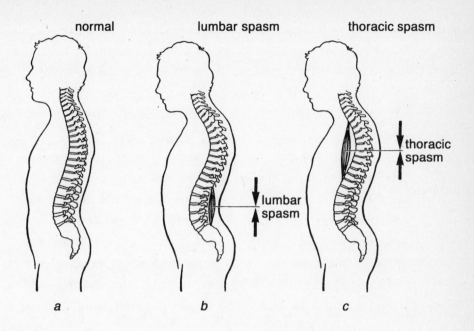

Figure 3.1 Diagram *a* shows a normal spine, with average posture. Diagram *b* indicates an increased curve in the lumbar region (lower back), caused by a spasm there. Diagram *c* illustrates an increased thoracic curve (upper back), caused by aspasm. Note how the curves in *b* and *c* cause the other curves to increase, as the body attempts to remain upright.

However, in poor posture some groups of muscles are stretched so when there is a rise in waste products and a lack of oxygen, these muscles will go into a cramp much earlier than they would have done if there had been better posture. Once the back has been treated and the muscle spasm reduced, posture will usually correct itself.

To illustrate this, look at the story of Arabella who, from the age of 12, was forced to try every trick in the book to correct her posture.

Arabella, then a 20-year-old student, was in absolute agony when she came to see me some years ago. Two weeks previously, she had lifted a television and felt a click in her back, and also suffered slight pain. The next morning she was in severe pain in the lumbar region, which did not respond to bed rest or anti-inflammatory drugs or painkillers.

When asked about any previous injuries, Arabella remembered falling off a swing at the age of eight and bruising her back. It recovered very rapidly, as so often happens in a child, and did not need treatment. Four years later, Arabella's parents and teachers started nagging her about her posture. She remembers walking with books on her head, practising endless stretching exercises and fighting a continual battle to keep her back straight. Her back started to ache at the age of 17 for no particular reason and this was put down to growing pains. She remembers vaguely that she lifted something fairly light and the next day felt some pain.

When standing, Arabella showed a marked increase in the curve of the thoracic spine (the section of the spine enclosed by the ribs). She was in too much pain to test movement but on palpation I could feel a severe spasm of the muscles on either side of the lumbar spine and this was present with decreasing intensity as far as her neck. It took 11 visits in all to get things right but by the end of the treatment she was altogether more comfortable. She also felt better in her general health and her posture improved considerably. After almost 14 years, Arabella has had no more back trouble. The nagging about her poor deportment has also stopped.

Not everyone is as fortunate as Arabella. In some cases, if the excessive curve has been present over a long period of time, the vertebrae can become wedge-shaped to accommodate it. Although the person is free from pain, a slight residual curve remains and becomes the normal posture.

The opposite situation to an increase in the back curve occurs if the muscles on the other side of the backbone produce the more powerful spasm. In this case, the pull of the muscles on the outside of the spinal curve will pull the curve flat, resulting in little or none of the original spinal curve.

*Does anxiety give rise to back problems?*

One of my patients once experienced the first agonizing pain in his back when he read a letter informing him that one of his companies had gone bust. He was keen to know if anxiety can cause back pain. What is the connection?

It is my belief that, in some cases where there is prolonged anxiety and tension, the continual pressure of the tensed muscles on the facet joints and the poor nutrition, caused by the consequent interference with the muscle pump, may bring about damage to the facet joints. Thus it is possible for prolonged stress to bring about back trouble in the absence of a pre-existing injury.

If a patient does have an underlying back problem, states of anxiety, tension, fright or excitement can be among the factors that produce pain. In some cases, they may even seem to be the only factors involved.

Although man has been variously civilized for probably 12,000 years, the fact remains that most of the physiological functions of the body still relate entirely to the primitive state. In those early times, anxiety was generally linked with physical danger, resulting in the subjective sensation that we call fright. This activates a special push-button mechanism called the sympathetic nervous system, which is associated with the adrenalin glands. The body is immediately put into a state of great efficiency for the suspected emergency.

The sensation of fear stimulates the system and the body reacts rather like a ship clearing the decks and getting the guns ready for a fight. In the case of the body, it may be flight rather than fight, but either way it must do all that is necessary to increase its chances of survival.

Those survival tactics include, among others, increasing body temperature through the muscle activity of trembling. Everything works better at a higher temperature. Think of a snake. Its muscle temperature depends on its environment – it hardly moves when cold but becomes a very quick-moving animal in the hot sunshine. All body functions improve at high temperatures – the pulse speeds up, blood pressure and blood sugar levels rise, and the blood is re-routed from the skin (which goes white) and stomach (causing butterflies) to the muscles and brain where it will be most required. In the context of back trouble, the appropriate muscles are put into an increased contraction, ready for action. This makes more work for the muscles and may result in a cramp. This series of fight-or-flight reactions especially apply to the upper muscles of the arm, shoulder girdle and thoracic spine. The lumbar muscles are also involved, but to a lesser extent.

In primitive conditions, the time element is minimal – you are either dinner yourself or you have to get your dinner in a relatively short space of time. It is all over very quickly. The sensation of fright or anxiety prepares the body for rapid and efficient action.

In contemporary times, we all suffer anxieties and tensions. They may not require the same urgent response as in primitive days, but they are forms of the same fear and the body automatically reacts. The reaction is much less intense but in our stressful lives it can continue for hours, days, weeks or even months. Under these conditions, the increased tension in the muscles can easily be the critical factor in turning a symptomless back into a painful one.

*Is back pain psychosomatic?*

While I do believe that anxiety and tension can be precipitating factors in the onset of back pain, I am convinced that back trouble is not psychosomatic. However, some patients, such as Judy whose story follows, have a mental problem they cannot face, and this may manifest itself in physical symptoms.

Judy came to me complaining of a very painful knee. Although it had been operated on twice, she said there'd been no improvement. I was not able to find any clinical signs to account for her problems and so I began to ask about any other worries or concerns. After a while she confided that she dreaded having sexual relations with her husband. An ideal excuse had presented itself when she banged her knee on a table six years before, and the pain gave her a substitute for a 'headache'.

As the years went by, her subconscious manufactured the pain for the escape it gave her. She wasn't aware she was doing it. She genuinely believed her knee was in a bad state. I referred her to a psychiatrist and once she faced up to the real problem, her pain vanished.

Judy's pain *was* psychosomatic. She couldn't cope with a problem and therefore resolved it by suffering physical symptoms. Many doctors believe that all non-specific back pain is psychosomatic. Patients are often told there is no actual physical cause for their pain and they come to me for a second opinion. On examination, I usually find the pain to be very real and sometimes wonder why the sufferers have not complained more.

The first thing Edna did when she walked into my consulting room was to hand me a letter from her doctor. The letter said that although Edna complained of pain between her shoulders and in the lumbar region, he could find nothing wrong. He said he was only allowing her to come to me because she had insisted so strongly. He stated that her main problem was psychological and that the best thing I could do was to endorse the need for her to go to the psychiatrist that he was recommending.

Edna, a 48-year-old secretary, told me that she had become increasingly tired and low over the last seven years, and that she had started suffering occasional aches in her upper back over this time – especially during and after typing. She had been having treatment with diet and antacids for indigestion for two and a half years, but each time this only gave relief for a few months.

In the last few months the pain had become worse and she was now experiencing a new pain around her left chest. She had had physiotherapy with heat massage and traction on and off for some time but this only gave temporary relief. Detailed investigation ruled out heart trouble and no apparent problem could be found, so I conducted my own examination.

During the consultation, Edna revealed that she had been involved in a bad fall on a skating rink 15 years before. I was therefore not surprised to find intense spasm of the muscles, which was particularly obvious in the mid to upper thoracic spine. My examination confirmed the physical nature of her problem and a very tender fourth thoracic vertebra pointed to the cause of the chest pain. After 14 sessions of treatment, Edna was altogether better.

By their very nature, psychosomatic complaints are designed to gain sympathy and attention, or to change the sufferer's way of life in some way for the better. Back pain, however, is generally greeted with laughter or boredom. A painful back is second only to a mother-in-law as a music-hall joke, and if people do not laugh when you complain of your pain, the chances are their eyes will glaze over as they stop listening after the first sentence. People do not feel sorry for back-pain sufferers and the pain certainly does nothing to improve a patient's way of life.

Out of the several thousand people I have seen with back problems, I have yet to meet one whose painful back is caused by psychological reasons.

## CASE PENDING

When a patient has a back problem brought about by accident or injury, the extreme stress that they are put through for possibly three years while litigation is pending produces a great increase in the protective spasm. This could well make a moderate back problem considerably worse by the time the case has been settled. It would benefit all involved if these cases could be settled in a much shorter time than is now the case.

I also believe that judges may be sadly misled by the fact that patients may undergo a considerable temporary improvement after the litigation is terminated as the tensional spasm lifts. This may lead to the completely erroneous opinion that the patient has been exaggerating the symptoms to obtain a better settlement.

*What is the effect of the weather?*

People may laugh when someone claims to be able to forecast a change in the weather by the state of his or her rheumatics. Yet the fact remains that many back-pain sufferers do actually feel less pain on warm, sunny days and in clear, mountainous climes. Why should weather have an effect?

It is a common assumption that when the air is humid, poor evaporation from the skin, lungs, nose and throat leads to an increase in total body fluid, which causes any already inflamed areas to become more swollen and, in the case of joints, more painful. This is a mistaken belief.

Humidity is not a factor in back pain. It is the state of electrical charge, or ionization, of the particles in the air that causes differences in the level of back pain. An ion is a charged particle of gas. In sunny weather the air is predominantly negatively charged. With wind and wet weather, the air becomes more positively charged. The body is unaffected by negatively charged particles, but a positive charge can cause trouble. In sunny weather, when the air is charged with negative ions, patients can cope with particles of pollen or dust that may cause an allergy. On wet and windy days, these same particles may incite an attack of asthma or hay fever.

When you breathe in positive ions, they pass through the lungs to the blood where they react on the platelets, causing them to secrete a substance called serotonin. It is the serotonin that increases any inflammation and this intensifies any aches or pains. It also makes people feel lethargic, headachy and depressed.

POSITIVELY OPPRESSIVE

Many people can predict an oncoming storm by the heavy atmosphere produced by a plethora of positive ions in the air. A few flashes of lightning restore the negative charge and, although the steaming humidity remains, people suddenly feel quite different. All the aches, pains and headaches go and everyone feels bright and alert.

Ionisers of a suitable type and adequate output can be of great help in the home or work place. One positioned in the output of an air-conditioning plant can cure the 'sick building syndrome'.

*Does weight or height influence back pain?*

When no definite cause of the pain is diagnosed, people will blame almost anything they can imagine. Weight and height are common scapegoats – 'I've been told it's because I'm too tall, too short, too fat, too thin' – but from my experience, these factors are rarely to blame.

Overweight people are often told that the excess poundage is the cause of their back problem, but this is not often the case. Many very overweight people have no trouble with their backs. However, if you already have a troublesome back, being overweight may aggravate the situation. The extra weight may alter the curve of the spine, thus stretching the muscles. It would also increase their workload and make a cramp more likely. Attacks of pain may occur more easily and with greater frequency.

It is possible that backpacks, which are often heavy compared with the strength of the person carrying them, may subject the facet joints to a load that, over a period of time, could damage them, initiating back pain.

Height is often thought to be a cause of back problems, especially in men. Many patients have been told that their backs are unstable because they are so tall and this is the cause of their pain. Similarly, several short, stocky men have been advised that their size makes them liable to back trouble.

---

BACK IN COURT

In one extraordinary case, a 6ft 2in tall woman had been in a car accident. The doctor assessing the extent of her injuries said that 50 per cent of her back problems were due to her height and this should be taken into account in reducing her claim. When asked to comment, I pointed out that in my practice there was little difference in the incidence of back trouble at different heights and that I regarded her height as irrelevant.

---

*Is there any connection between back pain and diet?*

A common precipitating factor in the onset of a muscle cramp is a deficiency of calcium. The patient often suffers from cramps in the muscles of the calf or feet while resting, especially at night. They can be so bad that the sufferer needs to climb out of bed and walk about to relieve the pain. Cramps are generally worse at night because of the slowing of arterial circulation. The lack of movement causes a decrease in oxygen supplied to the muscles and an increase in waste products. This precipitates a cramp. Calcium can be given by injection or by mouth to prevent these cramps and bring long-lasting improvement. Some other trace elements such as magnesium can also reduce cramps.

Salt deficiency is a common cause of muscle cramp, although not often in the back. A deficiency is usually due to excessive sweating in very hot weather or during a high level of physical activity (the problem is known as miner's cramp). The salt level in the body falls to an unacceptably low level and the muscles go into a violent cramp. This may occur in any muscle and is made worse by exercise. A drink containing salt will usually bring instant relief.

If all the muscles in the body are in a near state of cramp due to any of these deficiencies, it follows that the muscles in the back may well become painful under conditions that would not normally affect them.

*Could a food allergy lead to back pain?*

Food allergies can be a precipitating factor in the onset of a muscle cramp and pain. They are generally accepted as a cause of swollen joints, catarrh, fatigue and headaches, and I have noticed an occasional relationship between food and back pain. Indeed, I have referred several patients to food-allergy specialists to complement their treatment. Results have been most satisfactory.

The main allergic or sensitive condition that has an effect on the spine is a low-grade food allergy. We all know the acute type that occurs when you eat , say, strawberries and shortly afterwards your face and other parts of the body become swollen and may be covered in a rash. It is not this type of allergy but the lower grade allergy, or food intolerance as it is often called, that we are discussing here.

FOOD INTOLERANCE

This term was devised to avoid confusion between a full-blown allergy and sensitivity to certain foods. Common foods that are considered to cause intolerance in some people are coffee, milk and white flour. Food intolerance can have the direct effect of causing a build-up of oedema in the group of muscles associated with the shoulder blades and joints, collectively known as the shoulder girdle, making a painful cramp much more likely. Elimination of the offending food can have a marked effect on the onset of symptoms.

Food allergies are well covered in specialist books, or ask to be referred to a nutritionist.

*Do viral infections cause back pain?*

Viral infections seem to be more and more frequent and can sometimes be the cause of severe back pain. Many people, instead of catching a cold in the normal way, have a slight snuffle and then start to suffer pain in their backs. Often, they will show no obvious signs of a virus; usually they feel very tired or unwell and generally run down.

A viral infection gets into the bloodstream and travels all over the body. It settles in a muscle by entering the individual muscle fibres and multiplying there. This causes inflammation of the muscle and can lead to pain.

A virus can attack the muscles in a normal back and be severe enough to immobilize the patient. People with bad backs, however, have an increased blood supply to the inflamed area and, as the infection is carried in the blood, the back receives a disproportionate amount of the infection. Once the infection has gone, the back pain disappears and the back is usually left with no after-effects. Similarly, the increased level of activity caused by the infection on long-standing back trouble almost always reverts to the original level once the infection clears. Both the pain and the infection can be lessened with a short course of anti-inflammatory drugs.

*Is my back pain due to the menopause?*

Many women who are starting the menopause suffer aches and pains between the shoulders and in the lower part of the neck. This is caused by a deficiency of oestrins (female hormones) – normal at this time in a woman's reproductive cycle – which probably leads to an increase in the tissue fluids. Hormone replacement therapy (HRT), which replaces the body's lost hormones, can be most effective in ridding the patient of pain.

The other great advantage of HRT is that it acts to limit osteoporosis, or thinning of the bones. It is most distressing to see women in their seventies and eighties with badly curved thoracic spines that are clearly very painful. Every so often I see an unfortunate woman who has a vertebra that has collapsed, simply unable to withstand the weight of the body any longer. Their pain could easily have been prevented with HRT in their earlier years. Until a few years ago, it was hard to put the clock back to relieve such patients of their weakened bones. Now, fortunately, there are substances that can help the body restore calcium to the bones. Two of these are Etidronate (didronel) and Alendronate, which is somewhat more potent.

## AN ALTERNATIVE TO HRT

Salcitonin is a substance that helps to stop bone loss, and it is particularly useful for women who are unable or unwilling to take HRT. Some women react badly to HRT and are not realistically able to take it. Others fear the increased risk of hormone-related cancers. It is worth noting that almost all the research undertaken in this country has suggested there was no greater risk, though recent studies have indicated a slightly increased risk. Also, if a hormone-related cancer *is* stimulated by HRT, it is possible that it grows faster and so may be discovered earlier, before it has had any chance to spread.

In my experience, the advantages of HRT are that it usually greatly improves a patient's health and wellbeing and does a great deal to prevent the ravages of osteoporosis. A collapsed vertebra is very difficult to treat and usually results in prolonged and painful bed rest. Every woman must assess the pros and cons and decide for herself what course she wishes to take.

*How is my back affected in pregnancy?*

This is a very complex question as there are several conflicting forces at work in your body at this very special time. The drug cortisone was discovered when medical researchers began looking into why women suffering from diseases such as rheumatoid arthritis suddenly felt the condition improve when they became pregnant. It was put down to the fact that the suprarenal glands on top of the kidneys secreted a considerable increase of cortisone (so called because the cortex, or outer layer, of the gland secretes the substance). It is a hormone that has very powerful anti-inflammatory properties and helps the body minimise the effect of stress. This agent works throughout pregnancy, which will tend to make a chronic back better to the point of being symptomless.

After a while, however, the chemistry in the body changes in readiness for producing milk, and this results in a relative deficiency of calcium. Unfortunately, the lack of calcium makes the muscles more likely to go into cramp. Many an expectant mother suffers from cramps in her feet or calves at night, which is a typical manifestation of calcium shortage. The calcium deficiency affects the back muscles and makes them more sensitive so that back pain begins to be a possibility again.

Two more factors may cause back problems in later months. The first is that the extra weight of the baby causes awkward stresses and an increased curve of the lumbar spine. This may lead to cramps of a very painful nature in the affected muscles. The situation is made worse by the fact that the ligaments of the pelvis begin to soften to allow expansion at the time of birth. The back muscles must therefore work harder to maintain posture. This again leads to an increased tendency to cramp.

To avoid these problems in pregnancy it is important to keep the calcium in the body at an adequate level by including calcium-rich foods (milk, cheese, sardines, broccoli) in your diet or taking it as a supplement if necessary. During pregnancy, the body carries an increased quantity of fluid, thereby making oedema and circulation difficulties more likely. Exercises are important to keep the circulation in the back muscles working as efficiently as possible.

If an expectant mother is known to have a back problem, I find it best to give treatment after the second month of pregnancy as a precaution against trouble later on.

If the patient has a bad attack of pain in the last months of the pregnancy, treatment with surged faradism, ultrasonic waves and remobilization are safe (as long as the pregnancy is normal) and will almost always abolish the immediate pain. Ultrasonic waves are quite safe for the expectant mother. I usually suspend treatment at this point and suggest that it be resumed after the baby has been born.

Drugs should be avoided during pregnancy for although anti-inflammatory drugs are not thought to cause problems, they have not been proved to be safe.

Anthea, aged 27, came to see me when she was seven months pregnant, in agony with lower back pain. She had suffered backache of a minor nature for some years. She said it was painful if she sat for too long or after carrying heavy shopping or standing over a sink or cooker.

Soon after she became pregnant, her back felt altogether better and she had no pain at all. She was obviously delighted and thought that her back problem was over. However, at about the sixth month she began to have cramps in her feet, which would wake her up in the night. She often had to get out of bed to relieve them – and they were getting worse.

The day before I saw her she had been bending over to put a joint of lamb in the oven when she felt her back 'go'. The pain rapidly became agony and was not easing. I gave her some treatment that largely freed her of pain but the next morning she had a modest return of the pain so I repeated the treatment. She had no further pain but still came to me five months later, as recommended, and was treated eight more times until all the spasm had gone.

Anthea has had no more backache for five years. She had another baby 18 months after the first and was free of pain throughout the pregnancy.

# 4 BACK TO SPECIFICS

## Identifying pain associated with your back

There was a faith healer of Deal
Who said 'Although pain is not real
If I sit on a pin
And it punctures my skin
I dislike what I fancy I feel.'

So far, we have looked at the causes of back pain in a general way. In this chapter, the subject is tackled in more detail. Individual structures of the back and the part they play in producing pain are explained.

My father always held that 'nothing is as frightening as the unknown', pointing out that the best ghost stories do not give a detailed description of the ghost, leaving that to be supplied by the reader's own dark fears and anxieties. It is the same when patients are not given enough of the right kind of information about their complaints. That is why I feel it is so essential to lift the cloak of mystery from back pain and give sufferers an insight into their own particular problem. You should be able to identify your specific problem from the different types of back pain discussed here, and gain a better understanding of the cause of the pain. It is worth adding that I always encourage parents of children with back problems to include them in any discussion of the diagnosis and treatment.

## WORKING IN PARTNERSHIP

Knowledge of your back should give you confidence to seek medical help and to keep pushing for treatment until you find relief from the pain. I know from experience that a tremendous effort is often needed by patients to get doctors to recognize their condition. Doctors are not always the most tolerant people.

An embarrassing memory from my student days seems appropriate here. I was among a group of six new and nervous students gathered around an equally nervous and very frail middle-aged woman on our first day in a hospital's outpatients department. One of our number was singled out to question her. 'Well, have you found out what's wrong with her?' asked the Great Physician. 'She has a painful back,' answered the student. This seemed to be the sum total of information that he had managed to extract. Suddenly, Sir lost patience. 'I am a very busy doctor,' he boomed loudly, in front of the poor patient. 'She must not waste my time by coming to hospital complaining like this. All women have painful backs.'

For reasons that will be made clear throughout this book, I believe that doctors, physiotherapists and sufferers must take back pain more seriously than they currently do. Osteopaths and chiropractors already recognize that other problems can arise from back trouble although their understanding may not agree with that of the medical profession. Back-pain sufferers themselves need to realize this. Even if the attacks of pain are at prolonged intervals and do not seem all that severe, they must be dealt with, if only to avoid or get rid of these other problems.

It is important to work in partnership with your doctor, and not to put up with 'just the occasional back pain'.

## LUMBAR PAIN

This varies greatly. It can be a slight ache or an extremely severe pain in the small of the back. The onset can be gradual over a period of days or quite sudden. It may even start instantaneously, accompanied by a loud click when the back feels as if something has 'gone out'. All these are probably variations of the same mechanism.

In previous chapters we have looked at the effect of a spasm on the muscles in the back. The spasm, which has no symptoms, leads to a build-up of oedema in the tissue spaces, resulting in an increase in waste products and a lack of oxygen. When this condition reaches a critical state, the muscle goes into cramp. Anything that either increases the demand for oxygen or nutrients or further interferes with the action of the muscle pump helps take the condition of the muscle closer to crisis level.

Now, if a muscle is fairly near a cramp, then perhaps after a long car journey a few fibres of the muscle may well go into cramp and produce a slight ache. You have the feeling that you want to wriggle your back a little to help it. This is nature's way of telling you to work the muscle pump and improve circulation.

If the muscles are nearer to a crisis, many more fibres will go into cramp and the pain will be considerable worse. If all or nearly all the muscle goes into cramp, the pain is extremely severe and you may not be able to move. This same mechanism also accounts for pain higher up in the back.

### What causes the 'click'?

The precise cause of the clicking sound in joints, either at the limit of movement or when something goes wrong, is not known although there are several theories about it. Almost certainly, more than one mechanism is at work. One of them is thought to be the bursting of a gas bubble when a joint is suddenly compressed.

However, the click that we are concerned with occurs when a muscle goes into cramp. This often happens when you are making a considerable muscular effort such as bending forward to lift something heavy. As you straighten, a muscle on the verge of crisis may go into a sudden acute cramp accompanied by a click. This is not, as many people imagine, a vertebra or disc being displaced.

When the spine has an increased curve through bending or is being rotated by a twisting movement, the vertebrae are off-centre to one another, and their bony projections – the knobbly bones you can feel in your back (see figure 1.5 on page 6) – are not in the usual alignment. Now, as figure 4.1 shows, many of the muscles in the back taper into a thin wire-like tendon over much of their length. When a muscle suddenly goes into cramp on bending or twisting, one or more of these 'wires' may be directly on top of one of the bony projections. With the sudden tension of the cramp, it may catch on the projection and flick on to the distant or wrong side of it with a distinct click. While the muscle's tendon is stretched round this bone, it is very difficult for it to come out of cramp. We have seen that muscles resent being stretched for extended periods of time and this applies even more when they are already in cramp.

The agonizing pain can continue for a long time, usually somewhere between three days and three weeks until the muscle eventually becomes so fatigued that it relaxes and the tendon loosens, passing back over the bone. This allows the muscle to shorten and to come out of the cramp.

Someone with extreme back pain is often put to bed until it subsides. Bed rest has been considered a cure for so long it has become something of a habit with doctors. The medical benefits are rarely

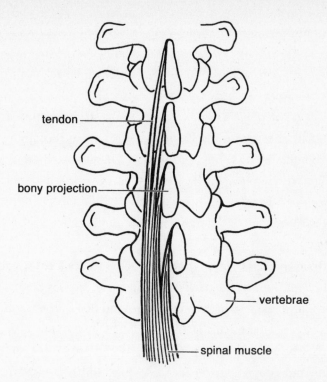

*Figure 4.1* Some of the spinal muscles raper to thin wire-like tendons. When the muscle is in cramp the tendon can easily slip and hook on to the wrong side of the bony projection.

either advocated or disputed. It is true that after some time in bed, a painful back nearly always feels better but, in fact, bed rest is of little positive help for back-pain sufferers.

As we have just noted, the pain will pass if you wait long enough for the muscle to weaken and relax, enabling it to free itself. After a certain time, your back will inevitably feel better, whether you are in bed or not. However, moving about as much as possible will speed up the recovery of the muscle from the cramp because the muscle pump is improved. Obviously, movement may be very limited but even a small amount will help.

Many people believe that if someone is in severe pain they should not be moved, but manipulation can often ease the pain. Manipulation at this stage effectively positions the back so the muscle tendon can untrap itself across the bony projection.

When treatment is successfully given to the stretched muscle, a loud click signals the release of the hooked-up tendon, accompanied by dramatic relief of the cramp and pain as the muscle shortens. People generally love to hear clicks when they are treated because they associate them with relief. It is commonly thought by the therapist that a displaced vertebra or disc has been 'put back'.

Richard travelled all the way from Bournemouth for a consultation, lying on a mattress in the back of his estate car. He was carried into the house and asked to be seen on the ground floor as he was in too much pain to attempt using the lift. I had just taken on a new assistant who was very experienced in the treatment of back problems and he agreed to see Richard while I finished with another patient.

When I returned, my new assistant had taken a history and done a quick examination.

'I'm afraid he's so bad he'll have to stay in bed for two or three weeks to improve enough to be treated,' he told me. I did not agree with this.

I explained that if we could free the trapped muscle, it would almost certainly come out of the cramp and revert to a symptomless state. Once I had tested Richard's back to see which way to manipulate him to untrap the muscle, I sat him on a stool and twisted him around. There was a loud click and the severe pain stopped immediately. He was left with a dull ache. After a course of treatment to relieve the basic spasm, Richard had no more back pain.

Why relief is temporary

I see a number of patients each year – such as Fred, whose story is below – who have been having bouts of pain every few months. Manipulation offers short-term relief by freeing up the muscle's tendon and is obviously of great value in stopping the pain, but it does not help the underlying condition. The time may eventually come when the muscle is so sensitive that it goes into a cramp even though it is not stretched. When this happens, the muscle is not necessarily trapped and manipulation offers little help.

It should be noted that, because muscles do not like being stretched, manipulation can sometimes cause a cramp but fortunately this seldom happens when a muscle is given a quick, sharp manipulation.

---

For about 14 years, Fred, a 38-year-old packer, had been prone to lumbar pain. The attacks were usually fairly slight but on occasion – once or twice a year – they became very painful. Initially, he was put to bed for up to a fortnight and each time the pain eventually went but came back later. Then he had physiotherapy, which helped a little.

Fred thought he had found the answer to his problem when he found an osteopath who gave him immediate relief from his pain. He continued to go for osteopathy once or twice a year, whenever he had an attack, for 10 years. Then, just five weeks before he came to see me, he said that for the first time the manipulation had not helped.

He had then tried heat, bed rest and traction but to no avail. He was very troubled when he was told that he had to have an operation on his back and was advised to consult me first. When I saw him he was a little better but still in some pain and he was worried about the future. He added that he tired easily, had slight indigestion and became momentarily dizzy on standing up.

When standing, Fred had an increase in the curve of the lumbar spine and there was considerable spasm of the back muscles from the upper thoracic to the lower lumbar region. After 11 sessions of treatment, he had no further trouble with his back and was amazed and delighted at his fast and permanent recovery.

## LOWER BACK PAIN

Trouble with the hip joints is a common reason for people complaining of lower back pain (below the lumbar region) usually on one side. Pain in the hip joint is generally felt in the buttock and sometimes slightly across the bottom of the back. There may also be pain in the groin. Pain may radiate down the back of the thigh to the knee and also from the groin obliquely down the front of the thigh to the inner side of the knee.

The hip joint is quite often overlooked as the cause. The diagnosis, however, is reasonably easy as movements that stretch the hip produce pain (see figure 1.12, on page 16). These movements include moving the leg out sideways, rotating the foot outwards or crossing your legs with knee across thigh.

### Sacro-iliac joints

You may remember from the earlier description that these are large, flattish bones that join the sacrum to the pelvic basin (see figure 1.12 on page 16). They are capable of little or no movement. A fairly severe blow may cause the ligaments that run across them to be stretched and many practitioners believe this allows one surface of the joint to slide on the other. As the surfaces are covered with irregular pits and humps (one side of the joint fitting exactly on to the other), it is thought that the joint may come to rest out of its true alignment.

The sacro-iliac joints are, in my experience, a relatively uncommon cause of pain in the lower back, except perhaps in pregnancy. Trouble in the sacro-iliac joints gives pain across the small of the back somewhat higher than the hip joint. The pain is usually on one side only. You feel pain if pressure is put directly on the joint or obliquely across the pelvis. This usually confirms the diagnosis.

Pain felt below the sacro-iliac joints is often due to the sacral one/two or three facet joints, and is best helped by anti-inflammatory injections.

## SHOULDER AND NECK PAIN

Fibrositic pains between the shoulders are usually cramps in the thoracic spinal muscles. Cramps may also occur in the bundles of muscles that run from the spine to the shoulders, under the shoulder blades. These cramps occur in muscles that are already in spasm due to bruising of the facet joints in the area. This causes the pain to radiate from the spine outwards underneath the shoulder blade to the actual joint.

Many women who are starting the menopause experience pains or aches between the shoulders and in the lower part of the neck due to a lack of oestrins, which probably increases tissue fluids. As mentioned in chapter 3, HRT can be extremely beneficial.

Polymyalgia (pain in a number of muscles) is another fairly rare cause of pain in the muscles of and across the shoulder joints.

A painful stiff neck is almost always due to cramp in the muscles of the neck. Sometimes the big muscles going from the trunk to the skull, especially the sterno-mastoid muscle, which pulls the ear and head down and forward, join in with the cramp. This is not only painful but may distort the head position.

A one-sided headache may well be caused by a cramp in one of the small muscles just below the skull. The pain can be very intense and of a migraine type. Pressure on the tender muscle often momentarily relieves pain.

## PAIN IN THE CENTRE OF THE SPINE

An inflamed supraspinous ligament is often the cause of pain in this area, and it can be difficult to treat. An anti-inflammatory injection often helps.

## REFERRED PAIN

Pains in the legs, arms, chest and other areas can be caused by back trouble. This is known as referred pain. The start of the problem is a nerve being irritated somewhere along the nerve's length. Far and away the most common cause of this is swelling of the facet joints. Other common causes include an inflamed hip joint that affects a nerve running nearby, a bulging or ruptured disc, a narrowing of the spinal canal (spinal stenosis) and tumours.

### Facet joints
As we have already seen, these joints can be bruised if the back receives a sharp jolt or suffers a jerking or twisting movement. Like any bruised joint, the facet joints may swell but normally there is enough space around them to accommodate the swelling without causing a problem.

If the joint has become acutely inflamed, however, it swells into the

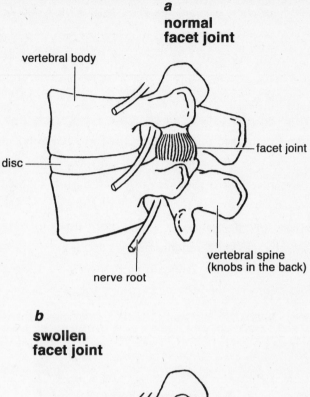

*a*
**normal
facet joint**

vertebral body

facet joint

disc

vertebral spine
(knobs in the back)

nerve root

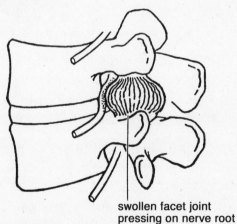

*b*
**swollen
facet joint**

swollen facet joint
pressing on nerve root

*Figure 4.2* Diagram *a* illustrates a normal facet joint, *b* shows a swollen facet joint.

neural canal and may touch or squeeze the nerve (see figure 4.2). As a result, you may feel referred pain in whatever part of the body the nerve supplies, usually the leg, quite often the arm and sometimes round the trunk. You may have pins-and-needles or other sensations rather than pain, and often there is numbness when the passage of sensory impulses along the nerve from the area is blocked.

Referred pain around the chest or in the abdomen usually occurs in people over the age of 40. If the pain is on the left side of the chest and/or down the left arm, it is very common for it to be mistaken for a coronary thrombosis, but when the chest pain is referred from the back, an electro-cardiogram is, of course, normal. Another distinction between the two is that a vertebra that is pinching a nerve has a very tender knobbly projection (the part of the spine that you feel when you run your fingers along the centre of the back).

It is rare for anyone under 20 to experience referred pain in the abdomen or chest. However, as this extraordinary story shows, it can occasionally occur.

In the early days of my practice, a lady telephoned me from Norfolk. She said that her seven-year-old child was suffering from a very painful tummy and the doctors did not seem to know the cause. The child had recently been in hospital for three weeks but no physical diagnosis had been made; the pain was thought to be psychological by the doctors. The mother was keen for a consultation but I explained that abdominal pain was not my speciality and recommended a paediatrician.

Imagine my surprise when she arrived in my consulting room three days later. I was even more bewildered when she explained why she was so sure I could help. Shortly after she had put the telephone down from our conversation it had rung again. This time it was a Mr Brown, who explained that he was a Norfolk witch and that his familiar had given him a message to pass on, the essence of which was that the source of the child's pain was in her back. The father made enquiries and found that the witch lived about 40 miles away and was well known for helping sick cattle in his area.

Although I could still see no possibility that the pain was anything other than some abdominal disorder, I examined the child. The abdomen appeared normal so I turned the child over and looked at her back. To my astonishment there was an area of acute protective spasm in the muscles of the back with a nerve that ran from the vertebrae to the exact spot where the child was complaining of pain.

Treatment to the child's back rapidly relieved the pain in her abdomen. I cannot pretend to say that I can explain this rather strange story but I just record it as fact.

## How can back trouble cause a painful calf or heel?

Referred pain is not easy to understand. To explain, let us compare the body to a hotel. Imagine you are in hotel room number 512. When you press the bell for room service, an indicator board will flash room 512 and the maid will know where to go to get her instructions. A similar process occurs in the body. A nerve ending is represented by the bell push and the indicator board is in the brain. The brain makes you aware that the origin of the sensation is at the actual point of stimulation, say the calf or the heel.

Now let us suppose that some careless carpenter drives a nail through the insulation of the wire somewhere on its path from the bell push to the indicator board. The flasher indicates that somebody is pushing the bell in 512 and the maid does not realize that the impulses originate partway down the wire.

In the same way, the brain thinks that the impulse originating from the neural canal in the spine is actually from the sensor at the nerve ending in the calf or heel and so registers the pain as being there (see figure 4.3).

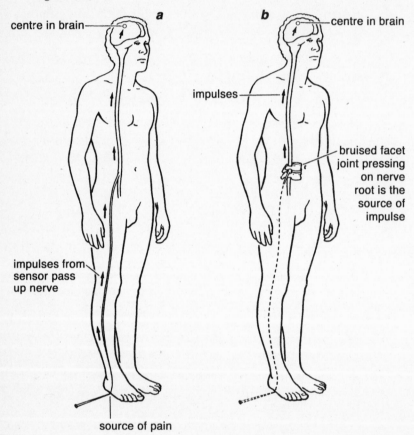

*Figure 4.3* In diagram *a*, the source of pain in the foot (e.g., a pin prick) sends impulses from a sensor, up the nerve to the centre in the brain, where it is registered. In diagram *b*, however, where a facet joint has swollen to pinch the nerve root from the foot, the impulses pass along that same nerve, to the same part of the brain, which registers that the pain is in the foot.

A nerve is like an electric cable with thousands of separate individual wires in one sheath. When it is squeezed, hundreds of nerve fibres are involved, all sending their impulses to the brain – which misinterprets them as coming from their appropriate nerve ends. A patient may, for example, feel a sensation of pain from the thigh right down the leg to the foot although the impulses actually originate from the one place where the nerve is being squeezed.

Incidentally, any pain in the sciatic nerve down the leg is called sciatica, whatever the cause may be.

### Spinal stenosis

Another more recently discovered cause of referred pain – especially in the neck and low lumbar regions – is a narrowing of the canal that runs through the vertebrae housing the spinal cord. In the neck region, this causes pain and stiffness and, more importantly, it causes pain to radiate across to a shoulder and down an arm, maybe to the fingers. In the lumbar spine, it causes a vague variety of pains in the hips, genital area, thighs and down the legs. The pain may go right down one leg but remain in the hip area of the other leg. Other sensations that may be present include a feeling of hot water being poured over the back of the legs and a very cold or very hot foot or feet.

Diagnosis can be made partly on symptoms but more accurately with an MRI scan (see page 82). At present the only effective treatment for this condition, when it becomes bad enough, is to hollow out the canal to restore it to normal size. Nerve conduction tests are also a great help in locating the exact site of the compression.

### The intervertebral disc

Although much maligned, in my experience intervertebral discs rarely cause problems. However, it is still worth considering what can go wrong.

As we have already seen, the disc is a flexible, circular, fibrous box with a flat top and bottom welded on to the vertebra above and the one below. It is full of an elastic jelly and behaves as if it was spongy rubber separating the two vertebrae. It has two functions. The obvious one is to allow movement in various planes between the two hard, flat vertebral faces but also it is part of the mechanism for absorbing the shock of a blow to the spine. It is a very strong structure and, in my view, is seldom damaged.

### What can go wrong with a disc?

The disc can be *compressed* as muscles in spasm put pressure on the adjacent vertebrae. If you imagine sitting on two tins with thick spongy rubber between, it is clear that under this pressure a disc may well bulge. If it bulges into the neural canal it may touch the nerve (see figure 4.4b). This will not cause pain from the disc itself but in the distribution of the nerve (see 'How can back trouble cause a painful calf or heel?'). Occasionally, the cramp of the muscles is felt as back pain but the intense referred pain is so overwhelming that this is hardly noticeable.

The condition is fairly easily corrected by treatment that relaxes the spasm of the muscles. The pressure is taken off the disc and it returns to a normal shape, thus relieving the pressure on the nerve.

The spinal cord is very large in diameter and occupies most of the space available in the canal. As a result, if a disc that is being compressed by the spasm bulges backwards, it can touch the spinal cord, resulting in impulses being sent up to the brain from the affected area (see figure 4.4c). This causes pain, not where the disc is – usually in the mid-chest area – but at the very base of the spine, and it may radiate into one thigh. When severe, the pain can be in the back, some way down one leg and in the other buttock.

The second and more serious cause of pain from a disc is when, as a result of prolonged pressure from the muscle spasm, the fibrous wall of the disc *ruptures* and the jelly pours out (see figure 4.4d). This tends to

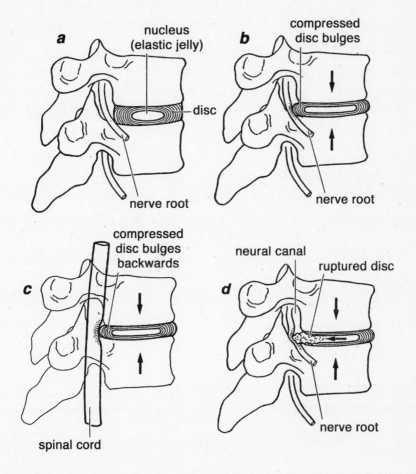

Figure 4.4 Intervertebral disc problems. Diagram *a* indicates a normal, healthy disc. Diagram *b* shows the compressed disk bulging sideways. Diagram *c* shows the same thing, but bulging backwards to the spinal cord. Diagram *d*, less frequent, is the result of a ruptured disc. Note how the contents of the disc (nucleus) have escaped, compressing the nerve root.

stretch the nearby nerve passing through the canal. The nerve is increasingly stretched as the jelly continues to flow out and, after it has been out of the disc for a while, begins to solidify. Although there is often little or no pain in that area, the inflamed nerve sends impulses to the brain, which again misinterprets them as coming from the beginning of the nerve.

In very rare cases, the fibrous wall may be ruptured by an acute injury, such as a fall from a height of over 15 feet.

If a disc has ruptured, the pain is severe and relentless. However, in my experience a disc lesion is comparatively rare.

### MRI (magnetic resonance imaging) scans

In the unlikely event of a disc being compressed or ruptured, it is usually in the lumbar region. Most patients feel pain in the sciatic nerve down the leg but it is also possible to feel pain in the foot, arm, round the body or in the chest, according to the positioning of the disc and nerve.

The actual location of the disc and the exact extent of the damage can be accurately imaged by an MRI scan. The equipment is an ingenious piece of apparatus that measures the bending of a powerful magnetic field by the fluids present in the body. As the amount of fluid in different tissues varies considerably, a detailed and accurate depiction of the tissues in relation to each other can be obtained. It images the discs and spinal canal as clearly as if the bones had been opened up and a photograph taken.

A test called a nerve conduction test is very useful as it plots the course of impulses in the nerves and shows if there is any break in their passage. This can accurately locate the spot where the nerves are being interfered with.

KEEP THE DISC!

When the MRI machine was first used, if a rupture of a disc was seen with a nerve wrapped round it, the only possible treatment was deemed to be removing the offending disc. This was therefore almost universally recommended.

My first shock came when my own doctor asked me to see him in the London Clinic. He had agonizing sciatica and was to have a disc removed the next morning. When I saw the absolutely massive disc on the MRI scan, I joined the other opinions concerning the necessity of its removal. He, however, had different ideas.

'I don't want an operation,' he said. 'I would like treatment.' I showed him the size of the disc once more and explained that it *had* to be removed.

'But,' he remonstrated, 'I've sent you dozens of people like this and you've managed to help them.' I pointed out that they had not had massive disc lesions. 'How do you know?' he countered. 'We didn't have scans to show it either way.'

He had treatment and an epidural (an anti-inflammatory injection into the space between the spinal cord complex and the bones of the spinal canal) and made a good recovery.

Two more patients convinced me that we had got it all wrong. Now, unless excessive pain or some neurological complication makes surgery obligatory, treatment usually wins.

I think what happens is that, with the pressure of the muscle spasm removed, the disc retreats back between the two vertebrae. The now hard jelly is dragged back by the rest of the disc so that it is more or less pulled off the nerve. White cells finish the job over a period of weeks by removing piecemeal anything of the extruded disc that is left.

## LOOKING AT THE UNDERLYING PROBLEM

Of the several hundred back-pain sufferers whom I see each year, on average only one has a ruptured disc. I have always felt that the disc is exaggerated as a cause of back problems. Too much research is devoted to the various attributes of the disc and not enough to what may actually be causing the problem.

You could say that it is rather like having a bus shelter that is continually being hit by a bus. Sophisticated research is directed towards finding the best materials to make a bus shelter strong enough to withstand the force and limit the damage. Endless statistics are compiled on the design of the shelter when all the time a simple tightening of a loose nut on the steering of the bus could solve the problem completely.

Many back problems do not cause symptoms that are directly associated with the back. Although you may not feel pain in the back itself, the underlying problem in the spinal column can affect nearby structures and systems and cause serious problems in other parts of the body. This often results in a number of well-known disorders not usually associated with the back, as well as a condition I have called hyposympathetic tone (HST). These will be considered in chapters 6, 7, 8 and 9.

# 5 YOUR BACK AND A HEALTHY SEX LIFE

## A good reason to have effective treatment for your back

Back trouble does not affect the development and functioning of the sexual apparatus. The development of the genitalia and their production of sperm or eggs are controlled by chemical messengers. These originate in the pituitary gland, which rests beneath the brain in the skull, and in the sex organs themselves – outside the effect of any back trouble.

The sex act, however, is a very different matter and can be affected in several ways by problems with the spine:

- directly, by pain in the back
- by interruption of the nerve supply to the area
- by low sympathetic drive

### PAIN IN THE BACK

Anyone who has a painful back knows that certain positions are out of the question – even adopting the gentlest of poses can prove agony. Muscles don't like being stretched and sex involves a lot of bending and stretching. For some men, that can create real problems.

Jack, 45, came to see me with general backache. He said that one of his problems was that he found twisting and bending forward most uncomfortable. He also mentioned that it was upsetting his sex life.

He had tried taking painkillers but these had damped down his sexual sensitivity and made the situation even worse.

The problem had started when he fell off a ladder a few years previously. Until then he had enjoyed a very good sex life and although his wife was very understanding, it was starting to cause tension between them.

Over the years I have come to realize that men are far less understanding of their partner's problems than women. Many women tell me that their backs are so painful they can take no active part in sex and even find lying still throughout intercourse almost unbearable. Yet their male partners all too often fail to show any understanding.

When Jane came to me she was suffering from lumbar trouble after a car accident in which she had been injured 10 years before. She explained that one of the most unfortunate results of this was that she went through some considerable pain every time her husband, Gary, made love to her. The pain was so severe when she moved that she rapidly learned to lie passively during intercourse.

Eventually, Gary became upset by this and started to get critical. His attitude, together with the pain, made Jane less enthusiastic about sex. Gary began to have premature ejaculations and poor erections. In the end, Jane was completely turned off.

Gary told her that he was working late more and more often until the day came when an emergency at home meant that she had to trace him. She found him in bed with another woman.

With correct treatment, Jane's back problem disappeared and her urge for sex returned. If only Gary had shown more sympathy and patience they could have continued to enjoy a happy marriage and fulfilling sex life together.

## INTERRUPTION OF NERVE SUPPLY

The sex act involves a complex interlinking of nerves that are situated at the lower end of the spinal cord. These are activated by both the brain and by sensory nerves that emanate from various erotic centres in the body. The most important of these by far are the cluster of nerves in the clitoris and parts of the vagina in women, and the tip of the penis in men. When stimulated, these nerve centres send impulses along the parasympathetic nerves to activate the sex organs. In the lumbar region, the parasympathetic nerves pass through the spinal nerve canal along the second, third and fourth lumbar nerve roots.

If back trouble has caused the facet joints, or even perhaps the intervertebral discs associated with these nerve roots, to become swollen, this may have serious repercussions. The swollen joints or discs will press on the nerve roots as they pass out between the vertebrae and may well inflame the nerves at this spot. This can result in an interruption of the passage of the impulses along the parasympathetic fibres from the spine to the genitalia causing three main problems:

■ **Blood vessels do not dilate**. This causes problems for both partners. An erection is brought about by impulses coming down from the back to the arteries, causing a sudden rush of blood. The blood vessels in the walls of the arteries dilate to allow this increased supply of fluid to fill the space, which is collapsed under normal circumstances, and it expands over the entire length of the penis thus giving rise to an erection. When the nerve supply is interrupted, the blood vessels do not dilate and men have a poor erection, or are not able to get one at all.

For women, in normal circumstances, the increased blood supply fills the cavities to enlarge the clitoris and to expand a ring at the entrance of the vagina. If the nerve supply is interrupted, this does not happen and women suffer from vaginal dryness. Although this is not quite such a catastrophe as the problem is for men, it still makes sex less enjoyable for both partners.

MORE PROBLEMS FOR WOMEN

An upset in the control of the blood supply to the uterus can lead to very heavy periods although it must be stressed that it is only when other causes have been eliminated that this should be considered. The increase in blood has another unfortunate effect – the liquid blood may clot because it has not been drained sufficiently rapidly from the very small tube of the uterus. These clots are removed, in the same way that a baby is expelled, by painful contractions.

■ **Little sensation**. If the sensory nerves are interfered with in any way, erotic sensations may be dulled for both men and women. This diminished sensation will result in men finding it hard to achieve an erection, and even if they do, it is almost impossible to reach a climax.

For women, it is not such an obvious problem but the same applies and this lack of satisfaction may dampen any enthusiasm for sex. The big difference is that with the man it is obvious to both partners and this can cause psychological problems in as much as his fear of being shown up can in itself cause impotence.

■ **Acute sensitivity**. If a nerve root is being compressed, even a light touch can give rise to pain in the part of the body it supplies. This can make sexual intercourse painful for both men and women.

In the normal course of events, if someone touches you lightly your nerve endings send a few impulses per second to your brain, which registers that you are being touched lightly. If you are being touched more firmly, the number of impulses per second increases to about 15 or so. When you are being pinched hard, the number rises to over 20 and your brain registers pain.

When the same nerve is being pinched halfway along its length, the situation changes. The pinched nerve sends back a steady 10 to 15 impulses per second from the affected area to the brain. The brain largely suppresses this information because the impulses arrive in a constant stream. However, if the nerve is touched and it sends back around 10 impulses per second, these impulses combine with the steady 10 to 15 to make over 20, which produces the sensation of pain.

In a situation where a person is suffering from compression of nerves in the back, these nerves are already sending the brain a high quota of impulses so it takes a small degree of sensation to turn touch into pain. This usually happens at the very last moment when the awareness of the sensation is at its height. Patients with back trouble complain of experiencing pain in the penis or vagina at exactly the wrong moment, making sex most uncomfortable. If this happens on several occasions, you will probably start to dread sex. For some men, the extra sensitivity triggers off premature ejaculation.

Guy, 32, had a lot of lumbar pain with some sciatica. An examination revealed a great deal of spasm in the muscles in the lumbar spine owing to considerable bruising of the facet joints. A course of treatment reduced the spasm considerably and, interestingly, he asked me whether the treatment could possibly be having any effect on his sex life. When I asked him to explain he said that for several years he had been having a lot of problems and had been seeing a counsellor. He said that he reached a climax as soon as he and his wife started to have sex. His wife was getting nothing out of it. However, things had improved dramatically since the treatment to his back and his sex life was virtually back to normal.

The reason for this turnaround was that before treatment, the nerves in his lumbar spine were compressed thus causing increased sensitivity. Once the pressure on them was reduced, the sensitivity also eased.

PAINFUL PERIODS

Hypersensitivity can be a cause of this distressing problem. The spasms of the muscles of the uterus often turn into mild cramps giving pain at the time of the period. In the same way that mild sensation can cause pain during sex, the discomfort or slight pain of the period becomes sharp pain for the sufferer.

■ **Low sympathetic drive.** As we will see in chapter 6, thoracic back trouble may lead to a condition I have called hyposympathetic tone, or HST for short. One of the main symptoms is excessive tiredness, which can lead to depression. This extreme fatigue is hardly conducive to an enthusiastic sex life and it is no wonder that patients often tell me they seek any excuse to get out of lovemaking with their partners.

Another symptom is a build-up of excessive acid in the stomach, which leads to problems with absorbing essential nutrients. One of the early casualties is Vitamin B. Lack of this vitamin adds to the problems of tiredness and inertia. It may also affect the ability of peripheral blood vessels to dilate, thus making it difficult to have an erection. Blood vessels not dilating also give rise to the problem of cold hands and feet – and, far less commonly, cold bottoms!

---

Alice, 36, had a problem with the whole of her back. She had aches between the shoulders and occasional attacks of lumbar problems with associated hip trouble. The pain was having a profound effect on her sex life to the point where she had almost given up.

She also complained that she felt tired all the time and seemed to lack any inclination to make love. But the biggest problem of all, she confessed, was that she had an ice-cold bottom that boyfriends found most off-putting.

Once her back was treated, all her problems melted away.

---

For Paula, 23, the excessive acid in her stomach caused another problem – continual nibbling in an effort to mop up the acidity.

Paula actually came to see me because she had a lot of aches between her shoulders. At the consultation she confessed that she was eating all the time which was the reason why she was more than three stone overweight. She explained that she felt so embarrassed to be seen in the nude that she avoided making love.

When her back was treated, this hungry episode vanished. When I last saw her at her check-up she was losing weight and feeling much more self-confident.

AMENORRHOEA

For several reasons, HST can cause periods to stop. If you are feeling generally unwell, your periods tend to be scanty or dry up. The problems of absorbing essential nutrients, explained above, can lead to a deficiency in vitamin B and iron, which causes the body to try to conserve blood by withdrawing the monthly blood loss.

An imbalance between the sympathetic and parasympathetic nervous systems (see page 102) can have the direct effect of limiting periods.

## Loss of libido

The nerve complex in the base of the spine is influenced, apart from the sensory impulses from the genitalia, by tracts coming down from the brain. These have a very powerful effect on the output of the parasympathetic centres controlling the immediate sexual response. An erection can often be achieved in a few seconds without the local stimulus from the genitalia, simply by the affect of thoughts, emotions, visual stimuli and odours.

Unfortunately, this can work both ways. Pain, whether in the back or the sexual organs, embarrassment and lack of confidence can inhibit both the desire to have sex and the act itself. If the act is unpleasant, the brain switches off the sexual urge as nature's way of finding an escape from a difficult or painful situation. This can eventually lead to impotence in men and frigidity in women.

Gladys, 42, came to see me because of back pain. She had fallen off a wall, flat on to her back, at the age of 17. Eight years later, she began to have low lumbar back pain. She had seen several practitioners but although she had been given immediate relief, the pain kept recurring.

Another problem, however, had gradually crept in and by the time she came to see me it had become a matter of the greatest concern. She had had pain so often when making love to her husband that she had begun to lose all interest. She had no desire for sex at all. This was having such a bad effect on her husband that she told me her marriage was heading for the rocks. Fortunately, things were not irretrievable and as her back recovered, her participation and enjoyment in lovemaking resumed.

If you are feeling below par, the brain will turn off your desire for sex. The law of survival of the fittest means that anyone in a poor state of health isn't fit to have a baby. If you are feeling tired or depressed, you probably wouldn't want one anyway. So nature responds with a powerful turning-off effect for both men and women in an attempt to exclude conception. This has a greater influence on women than on men but it is not unknown for a man to become impotent under these circumstances, which is an altogether more dramatic result.

Clive, 37, had fallen off his motorbike nine years before he came to see me. He had some backache, mostly between the shoulders, if he drove any distance or if he used his arms too vigorously. He tired very easily and had indigestion for which he was being treated. He had also had two minor depressions during the last three years.

Clive needed 11 visits to get rid of the spasm in his back and alleviate all the other associated complaints. It was not until near the end of treatment that he began to enjoy a most unexpected and positive effect on his sex life.

For two or three years previously he had become progressively less interested in lovemaking and more recently he had even been impotent on a few occasions. As he lost confidence, the problem got worse. Now, for the last two or three weeks, there had been a remarkable change. His interest and desire had returned and he was having no more problems with getting an erection.

There is so much psychology involved with sex. If you feel under pressure, or are simply anxious to please your partner, even if you desperately want sex, the whole episode can prove disastrous. One failure can lead to another and a complete breakdown in confidence often follows. Sex is an important part of a happy relationship. I have seen all too many marriages come apart because of the difficulties one partner finds in having sex. This must be one of the most compelling reasons for having effective treatment for a bad back, whether or not the back is painful.

Of course, treatment to the back does not hold the key to every sex problem. However, when all other possibilities have been investigated without success, a back problem should be considered.

# 6 BACK TO FRONT

## Your back problem and a common new disease

> Patient: 'I hope you will find that I am ill.'
> Doctor: 'What do you want to be ill for?'
> Patient: 'I would hate to be well and feel as I do.'

People often come to me saying they feel unwell without being able to pinpoint the real cause. Tiredness, depression, indigestion, dizzy spells and headaches, together with a feeling of being 'not quite right' are common symptoms. Many of these people have been given treatment for one or more of the symptoms individually but often they say that it has had no lasting effect.

Given these symptoms, a full investigation is obviously necessary and a very important part of that is to examine the person's back. It is my firm belief that if none of the better-known causes have been found, the back is usually the source of the problem. I find that once the back is treated, the illness also clears up. The back may either have no symptoms or be painful – in either case people seldom connect it to all the other symptoms. Treatment of the symptoms alone does nothing to cure the overall trouble. It is a sad fact that tens of thousands of people are suffering with little hope of finding an answer to their problems.

The story of a prominent businessman who came to see me some years ago illustrates the point. I diagnosed the cause of his symptoms as silent back trouble and after several treatment sessions he was back on top form.

Lord D, a well-known workaholic, complained that recently he had started to feel excessively tired and, at times, very depressed. He also had difficulty in concentrating and was beginning to fight shy of anything that was likely to put him under pressure. He told me that he had been to see his GP and asked to be referred to a top consultant to find out what was wrong. He had been in a nursing home for three weeks. All his body fluids had been analysed, he had been X-rayed and scopes had been inserted through every orifice possible.

Eventually, Lord D found himself sitting in front of the consultant, who had a pile of test results, inches high, on his desk. The doctor tapped his knees and ankles and listened to his chest then said, 'I am very happy to tell you that there is absolutely nothing wrong with you at all.' Well aware that Lord D's name often appeared in the paper connected with takeover bids, he added, 'When did you last take a holiday?'

Lord D confessed that it was probably five or six years since he had really had a break. Convinced by the doctor that this was the cause of the problem, Lord D packed his bags and spent three months on a restful holiday in the South of France.

The holiday did little to relieve the symptoms and so Lord D asked to be referred for another opinion. This consultant looked through the large pile of tests that had been done, tapped his knees and ankles and listened to his chest and said there was absolutely nothing wrong. He continued by asking, 'What have you been doing with yourself recently?' When Lord D told him that he had been in the South of France for three months the immediate reply was, 'Well, all that's wrong with you is that you need a jolly good job of work.'

In many instances, the doctors may have been right to recommend a change in routine to help relieve the mysterious symptoms. However, there are also many people like Lord D for whom an examination of the back provides the necessary clues to the problem. Lord D was suffering from this common complaint that is, fortunately, usually easy to correct.

Before looking at this condition in more detail, let's examine the role tissue fluids play in the body because this is crucial to understanding the problem.

## EFFECTS OF A POOR MUSCLE PUMP

We have seen how a damaged or bruised facet joint causes a protective spasm of the muscles lying across it. This spasm, because of the pressure it exerts on the joint, maintains the bruising and thus the problem in the back is self-perpetuating. Under these conditions there may well eventually be symptoms in the back itself, usually pain.

The problem, however, may spread further than the spine and cause a number of other ailments. The blame for this lies with the diminished activity of the muscle pump, which results from the muscle being in spasm.

As noted in chapter 1, when a muscle contracts it compresses not only its own tissues but also the adjacent tissues, squeezing fluid and blood from them. Apart from those areas affected by gravity, this is the body's main mechanism for taking blood from the tissues and returning it to the heart. If spasm causes the muscle pump to work poorly, this pumping action is slowed down.

Earlier we looked at the effect of this reduced pumping on the tissues of the back muscles. Now let's see how it affects the adjacent tissues. One of the most important of these is the sympathetic nerve chain, which lies close to the spinal muscles in the lower neck and upper thoracic part of the spine. It is one of three separate but interdependent nerve systems in the body – the central, sympathetic and parasympathetic nervous systems.

- **The central nervous system** is the most important. It is dominated by the brain and includes the ordinary sensory and motor nerves that run around the body (see figure 6.1). The central nervous system controls all voluntary actions and all conscious sensations such as vision, taste and smell, hearing, skin sensations, muscle, joint and tendon status, and the pain of internal malfunctions, such as an injury or appendicitis.

- **The sympathetic nervous system** (see figure 6.2) is made up of a chain of nerve centres, called ganglia, connected to each other, to the spinal nerves and to virtually every part of the body. It influences the running of the entire body machine and monitors and controls a vast number of functions, such as blood pressure, blood chemistry and repair. It is also responsible for the body's built-in response in emergency situations.

- **The parasympathetic nervous system** consists largely of a nerve centre in the brain and a long nerve called the vagus (meaning wandering) that wanders all over the body (see figure 6.4). Also known as the vegetative system, it mainly controls the digestive tract, and its stimulation causes secretion of digestive juices and the churning movement of the stomach and bowel after

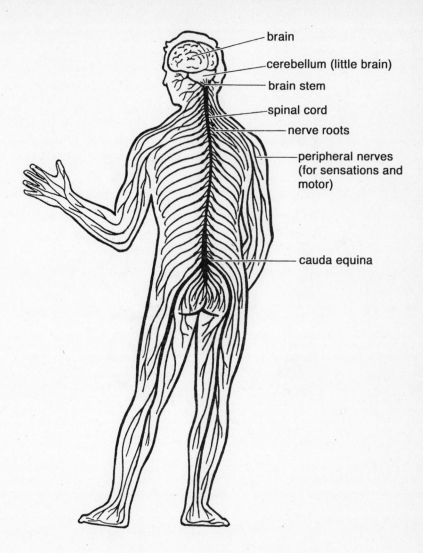

brain
cerebellum (little brain)
brain stem
spinal cord
nerve roots
peripheral nerves
(for sensations and
motor)

cauda equina

*Figure 6.1* The central nervous system, which runs throughout the whole body.

the intake of food. It works by having largely the opposite effect of
the sympathetic nervous system throughout most of the body – an
upset to one affects the other.

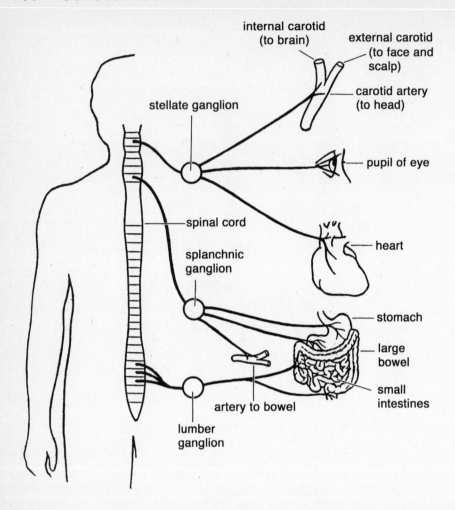

internal carotid
(to brain)

external carotid
(to face and
scalp)

carotid artery
(to head)

stellate ganglion

pupil of eye

spinal cord

heart

splanchnic
ganglion

stomach

large
bowel

small
intestines

artery to bowel

lumber
ganglion

*Figure 6.2* The sympathetic nervous system. The nerve centres (ganglia) are linked to specific organs in the body, and these are the organs which are adversely affected when the sympathetic nervous system is under pressure.

### The sympathetic nervous system

Why the name 'sympathetic'? It is from the French word *sympathique*, as this system was named by a Frenchman after he noticed that it caused an increased heartbeat in an emotional situation. In reality, this

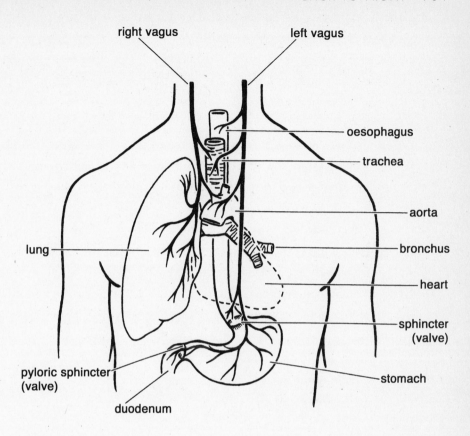

Figure 6.4 The vagus nerve (right and left) runs throughout the body, parallel to the sympathetic nervous system. It is the mainstay of the parasympathetic nervous system and we can blame the vagus nerve for excessive fatigue.

is because it is part of the adrenalin mechanism designed to put the body into a state of efficiency in an emergency, as discussed in chapter 3. In primitive conditions, this kind of emergency would be a purely physical one. The sympathetic nervous system prepares the body for instant and intense action. As it does so, you will experience:

- a rise in pulse and blood pressure
- repeated small contractions of a number of muscles, or trembling, which generates heat to increase body temperature
- sweating to prepare the skin for cooling during supreme physical effort
- an uncomfortable feeling in the stomach and a pallor in the skin as the blood vessels contract to redirect blood from areas where it is not required to areas, such as the muscles and brain, where it may be urgently needed
- head and body hair standing on end (think of a lion's mane or cat's fur) as possible protection against the teeth of the attacker and also convey greater size to frighten off the enemy
- shedding of unnecessary weight – or the first stage of shedding it when you feel sick, want to urinate and possibly want to defecate
- dilation of the pupils of the eyes to let in more light
- widening of the coronary arteries of the heart to allow for a sudden increased output
- the sensation of fright

In figure 6.2 you can see that different parts of the sympathetic nervous system along the spine affect various organs of the body. It is easy to see how the responses above would be experienced when this nervous system goes into action. Later we'll see what happens when it malfunctions.

Figure 6.3 shows some of the sympathetic nerve centres, or ganglia, in the neck, and indicates the large number of muscles surrounding them. It is clear how tensing these muscles would affect those ganglia.

Tug-of-war situation

In a healthy body, the sympathetic and parasympathetic nervous

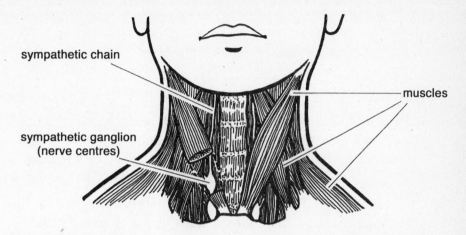

sympathetic chain

muscles

sympathetic ganglion
(nerve centres)

Figure 6.3 The sympathetic nerve chain lies close to the base of the neck. Note the large number of muscles surround it.

systems work in opposition to each other rather like two tug-of-war teams pulling equally against each other. Both nerve systems put out a continuous stream of impulses, which normally neutralize one another.

As in a tug-of-war contest, this equilibrium is disturbed when the output of one nerve system is increased or decreased. If, for example, something were to diminish the effect of the sympathetic nervous system, the normal pull of the parasympathetic previously neutralized would make it active. As the sympathetic nervous system slows down, the parasympathetic becomes dominant.

Under normal conditions, if one nerve system is stimulated, the other almost switches off. When, for example, the sympathetic system is activated through fear, the parasympathetic has little output so that energy is not wasted during the crisis by, say, the continuation of digestion. If the crisis (such as a fight) lasts only a few minutes, as it would have done in primitive times, this does not lead to problems.

However, if anything (such as business or domestic worries) causes a prolonged imbalance, this can have far-reaching effects on the normal functioning of the body.

### How a muscle spasm upsets the balance

The parasympathetic nervous system's main controlling centre is in the brain stem. This means that it is well protected and unlikely to malfunction, as it is unaffected by any outside influence. By contrast, the sympathetic ganglia, of which there are a number, are positioned near the muscles of the back, mainly in the chest area but also in the mid-lumbar region. They are far more at risk of being adversely affected by neighbouring conditions.

We have seen in previous chapters that when the muscles in the back are in spasm the adjoining tissues become waterlogged and this would, of course, affect any nerve centre in the area. If all the ganglia were affected by the congestion, the whole sympathetic activity, or drive as it is called, would diminish.

Each ganglion is a small mass of nerve tissue made up of millions of cells and their nerve branches – one of the 'mini brains' of the nerve system. Information from sensors travels along a nerve into the ganglion and arrives at a gap between that nerve and another nerve cell. It is passed to, or blocked from, the next nerve by chemicals, which are generated by other nerves that control the transmission.

The effect of a large chain of such reactions results in appropriate correcting messages being sent to the tissues concerned. This may well also be affected by information from other sources. Look again at figure 6.2 to see how each of the ganglia of the sympathetic nerve system supplies various parts of the body. The chemical control of the impulses is easily upset by excessive fluid in a ganglion.

When the sympathetic drive has been slowed down, the vagus

nerve supplying the same area, being relatively unopposed, displays excessive activity. Someone in this situation would have symptoms both of a low sympathetic drive and of extra activity of the vagus (see page 102). This combination of symptoms and signs results in the syndrome I have named hyposympathetic tone (HST), hypo meaning low or below normal.

## HYPOSYMPATHETIC TONE

HST affects a very large number of people and can, when severe, cause considerable distress and incapacity. Fortunately, it is readily diagnosed and can successfully be treated. The symptoms fall into four main groups:

- effects of a low sympathetic drive
- effects of parasympathetic over-activity
- compensatory reactions of the brain
- thoracic and lower neck trouble

### Effects of a low sympathetic drive
*Extreme tiredness* is usually the first and only symptom for several years. This is especially noticeable if life is smooth with no challenges. Pressure situations such as decisions at work raise the sympathetic drive and help to override the tiredness. However, once the pressure is off, the sufferer usually flakes out. After a time, someone with a low sympathetic drive may feel not only tired but also unwell. Sometimes they can become seriously ill.

The young are not immune to the condition, as the following case illustrates.

Jonathan was only 16 when he came to see me. Two years previously he had felt extremely tired for three months. Despite intensive investigations no reason was found and it was put down to a poor diet and pressure at school. He improved spontaneously and went back to his normal life. Six months before I saw him he suddenly became very tired again for no apparent reason. He said he felt like going to bed nearly all the time. He started to have momentary dizzy or faint feelings if he stood up suddenly. He was also extremely tense and had moments when he felt depressed.

It turned out that he had fallen off a horse six years earlier and had landed on the back of his shoulders. When I examined him, I found a spasm of the spinal muscles – caused by the old injury to his thoracic spine, which had bruised the facet joints – stretching from the neck to the low thoracic region, plus an increase in the thoracic curve. The spasm of the muscles had caused oedema in the area and this had depressed the sympathetic nervous system, causing tiredness. Dizziness was caused by ensuing momentary falls in blood pressure.

I treated him with physiotherapy and manipulation of his thoracic spine but Jonathan's problem took a long time to cure. Although he felt vastly better after six visits, he kept relapsing a little and needed more treatment. Finally, after 28 visits over one and half years he was well and stayed well.

Tiredness caused by a low sympathetic drive has certain distinct characteristics. It seems to peak at around three or four in the afternoon after which you may perk up again. A short rest may be all that's needed to overcome the tiredness. Indeed, it seems that excessive tiredness at any time of the day can be relieved by a rest or sleep of as little as five or 10 minutes. The other characteristic is that there is an inversion of the sleep mechanism – you sleep badly at night and are tired all through the day.

Restful holidays are often recommended to sufferers but they are not a great success for anyone with HST. As mentioned above, the sympathetic nervous system needs a challenge to maintain a reasonable level of drive and so a restful holiday is seldom helpful. Even if it is, it is quite common to go right back to square one a few weeks after returning and to feel that you might just as well not have gone away.

*Low blood sugar* is another symptom of a low sympathetic drive. This may happen periodically, making patients feel weak and cold, sometimes with a clammy sweat. They may also experience a sense of unease, even a feeling of impending doom.

*Low blood pressure* is another common sign. In most cases it is very much at the lower end of what is usually regarded as normal. Patients often say their blood pressure has been rather low for a number of years but they were not aware that it was a problem. Common effects of low blood pressure are dizzy spells and a faint feeling when you stand up suddenly, especially after having been lying down.

For someone in late middle age who has had the problem for years, the blood pressure often begins to rise suddenly and tends to become excessively high. It may need treatment to lower it to within normal limits.

Effects of parasympathetic over-activity

- **Indigestion** in some form is a very common symptom. The high level of acid in the stomach inflames the lining, making it sensitive although the effect may be fairly mild. Often patients say that they cannot stop nibbling, which is nature's way of mopping up the excess acid in the stomach caused by the activity of the para-sympathetic nervous system, and they tend to be short of vitamins and trace elements (see page 127).

Some people lose their appetite if the lining is more inflamed because their stomach feels uncomfortable when they eat, and they complain of frequent belching. This is caused by the subconscious swallowing of air in an effort to separate the sensitive walls of the stomach, and it can be very difficult to persuade people that they are not in fact bringing up the air.

If the condition worsens, feelings of a lead weight or pain in the stomach may occur. In extreme circumstances, a gastric or duodenal ulcer may result. In this case, you will lose weight and find it almost impossible to put it back on.

■ **Putting on weight** is another sign of an over-active para-sympathetic nervous system. Dieting is virtually impossible if there is a compulsion to eat to keep the acid levels down.

About half the patients I have seen who have had a whiplash injury put on a great deal of weight. This causes distress and is yet another reason why they feel unhappy about themselves. These patients also tend to be short of vitamins and trace elements.

■ **Allergic reaction** may occur as the inflamed stomach becomes unusually sensitive to irritating foods. If this happens, it will sometimes activate the early warning system in the body that enables tissues to recognize a minute trace of a substance that has caused trouble previously.

It is rather like an army that has on a number of occasions suffered a full-scale assault by the enemy, preceded by the sighting of a few patrols. When a patrol wearing the recognizable uniform of the aggressor shows itself, an immediate full-scale mobilization takes place, even though the enemy army is on this occasion not present. In the same way, the body will react in a normal manner to this known irritant, but at a level that is excessively and totally out of proportion to the very small amount of it present.

These allergies usually regress as the stomach improves with treatment to the protective spasm in the back muscles. Occasionally, however, they do need treating in their own right.

## Compensatory reactions of the brain

■ **Tension** is often a dominant symptom of HST. Imagine the voltage is down in an all-electric house. You have no idea that the voltage is low but you do notice that the lights are a bit dim and that the cooker does not get as hot as it should. The washing machine is not working well, nor is the television or hi-fi. You call in specialists to test each individual appliance but no one can find anything wrong.

In the same way, doctors trying to diagnose someone with HST may find that each individual system appears to be normal. The filaments in the light bulbs are intact and of the correct resistance. The cooker heater elements are normal and the thermostats are all in working order. Naturally, you are left wondering whether you are imagining things.

However, if the specialists had looked beyond the working of the appliances to the voltage coming into the house, they would have found the reason for the inefficiency.

Fortunately, the body has sensors, which alert the brain to the fact that the sympathetic drive is low. Just like the house owner who is tired of the poor-working electric appliances, so the brain gets fed up with the unsatisfactory running conditions in the body and resolves to do something to correct things.

As we have already seen, when someone has had a shock, the anxiety/fright centre stimulates the ganglia increasing the drive. When the sympathetic nervous system is flagging, the brain tries to perk it up by simulating an anxiety and thus activating the anxiety/fright centre. This results in the patient becoming very tensed up. Most people think that being tensed up causes stomach and other problems when, in fact, they are both the result of the same illness.

■ **Sleep inversion** has already been discussed (see page 107).

■ **Depression** has many causes but it can also be one of the symptoms of HST. If someone has no apparent worries, or has a depressive personality, the tensed-up state can lead to attacks of depression that may be serious enough for them to consult a psychiatrist.

■ **A tense state of mind** is a mild version of fright but the body has a physical reaction designed to meet a crisis in the jungle. Among the effects of this emergency response, the muscles of the shoulder girdle and thoracic spine tense up ready for the impending battle. This further interferes with the muscle pump and so further aggravates the malfunction of the ganglia (see page 98). Under these conditions, you may feel even more tensed up and a limited vicious circle is set up.

■ **Inability to cope with a change in routine** is another classic symptom. You may find it hard to cope with events outside your everyday experience. This is because the subconscious brain, realizing that the defence mechanism is not working properly, tries to stop you going out of the cave. It suspects that if you were to meet a wild animal, you might not – without the benefit of a sympathetic boost – be able to cope with it. Even an invitation to be sociable with friends could seem too daunting and all sorts of excuses are conjured up in an attempt to avoid something that appears to the subconscious to be an impending confrontation. In reality, the best possible thing to do is to go to the social event. As soon as you arrive, you will see there is no danger and can then enjoy yourself.

Some while ago, Stephen was practically frog-marched in for a consultation by two concerned friends. Ten years previously he had started to feel rather tired and although he was normally very sociable, he had gradually become more and more reluctant to go out. As time passed, modest reluctance turned into marked reticence and he became quite anti-social.

Stephen's friends became alarmed when he started taking mornings and then days off work because he felt too tired to go in or said that he could not cope with events at the time. Before long, it got so bad that he rarely left his home. The final straw for his friends came when he started asking for food to be sent up to his room as he found it altogether too much to go downstairs to eat.

Stephen had seen a psychiatrist a few years before who said that he was somewhat depressed and needed a holiday. The holiday had done him no good and the feeling of inertia had gradually increased. When I asked him about any back trouble he seemed puzzled but revealed that he had had intermittent neck trouble and pains between his shoulders for many years. It transpired that about 15 years earlier he had been involved in a car accident, when he had suffered a whiplash injury.

On examination, it was clear that his sympathetic nerve centres had become involved when the facet joints were bruised by the injury, and had become waterlogged. The brain had over-reacted in its endeavour to increase the sympathetic drive. Once the back was treated he started to feel his old self again.

Thoracic and lower neck trouble

We have already seen how back trouble in the thoracic and lower neck areas of the spine can depress the activity of the sympathetic nerve ganglia, which lie close to the affected muscles. It follows then that a symptom of HST may be pain in these parts. Patients often complain of fibrositic (inflammation of the fibrous tissue of the muscle sheaths) or non-arthritic pain between the shoulders and/or base of the neck. On examination there is usually considerable spasm of the paravertebral muscles in the area.

Is there a cure for HST?

By healing the trouble causing the imbalance between the sympathetic and parasympathetic nervous systems, the harmony between the two can be restored and the various symptoms of HST will disappear. The treatments detailed in chapter 10 have restored the good health of the majority of sufferers who have been to see me.

FROM A GRATEFUL PATIENT

19 April 1990

Dear Dr Sherwood,
Having given my wayward and utterly unsympathetic autonomic ganglia a good airing recently in Texas, I thought that I must write

and thank you for what seems to me a miracle cure. While perhaps to you the treatment is routine, with no surprises, from my side of the ganglia it was a remarkable transformation, for which I am profoundly grateful.

Such is my confidence in you that when I come to see you in June for a 60,000 mile service I shall expect you to press the right button to effect an instantaneous cure for smoking. I feel sure that this must be within your expertise.

With warmest regards and renewed thanks,

PJ

## OTHER BACK-RELATED DISEASES

HST involves the whole sympathetic nervous system but it is far more common for just one or two centres to be affected by back trouble. Symptoms such as migraine and indigestion can of course occur on their own and are recognized as separate complaints. However, the way these problems have cleared up when the associated part of the back has been put right leads me to believe that a number of people who suffer from them have a partial sympathetic imbalance as their primary problem. This will be discussed in detail in chapter 8.

# 7 YOUR BACK AND ME

## Why ME is not such a mysterious disease

The disease known as ME has been given a variety of names including Icelandic disease, after the country where it was originally diagnosed, and Royal Free disease, after the hospital where the first recognized outbreak occurred in Britain. Post-viral syndrome is another common name and, although far from perfect, that is the one I prefer because, as a syndrome, it covers those cases that are obviously associated with an infection.

The name myalgic encephalomyelitis (ME) seems less satisfactory to me for several reasons that will become clear throughout this chapter. Firstly, I doubt whether the encephalon – the brain – is often, if ever, involved in the disease except in cases of extreme severity. Secondly, myalgia – meaning a number of painful muscles – is usually ascertained by an erythrocyte sedimentation rate (ESR) test, which measures the settling properties of red cells in the blood. This is calculated by placing blood in a vertical tube and observing the quantity of red cells that settle in the bottom of the tube after an hour. Curiously, this is a very sensitive measure of the degree of activity of the defence mechanism when the body is responding to either an inflammatory or an infectious disease. A raised test result under these conditions usually indicates polymyalgia. In patients suffering from ME, the ESR remains normal, as do most other tests.

## A POORLY UNDERSTOOD DISEASE

There is a great deal of confusion about ME – indeed, some doctors believe it is simply a figment of the imagination. People suffering from similar illnesses are often classed as ME patients and this makes it difficult to integrate the signs and symptoms into a single disease.

One form of it can occur at the same time as a very severe attack of one of a number of common virus infections. Most patients who have this particular problem are treated in specialized units. It is a grave condition and quite rare, and is not typical of the disease affecting the majority of sufferers.

An inflammation of the brain and spinal cord (encephalomyelitis) is thought to cause a number of the symptoms found in ME. These include tiredness, depression, muscle weakness and pain, plus sensory symptoms such as pins and needles. There are, however, much simpler alternative explanations for these symptoms, which are discussed in this chapter.

To shed some light on the matter, let us look more closely at the particular disease that I prefer to call the post-viral syndrome. Many of the symptoms were apparent in a 55-year-old bank manager who came to see me recently.

Joe had been feeling very slightly off-colour for several years but he put it down to the onset of old age. Five years before he came to see me, he had suffered an attack of influenza and was left feeling very tired and depressed for several weeks. After about six months he had flu-like symptoms again, followed by depression and, more distressing, a feeling of complete exhaustion. He had only to do the slightest thing such as get up and walk in the garden and he felt completely knocked out and had to go to bed for at least 24 hours.

Joe had further slight flu-like attacks every few months for about a year. Just as he was starting to feel better, he would be hit by the symptoms again. He started to feel pains in his legs, especially the left, and they became very heavy. He also had aches in his neck and shoulders and suffered mild indigestion. A more constant and, to Joe, more worrying symptom was a woolly feeling in his head, lack of concentration and an obvious slowness of thought.

When Joe came to see me he had been unable to work for about two and a half years. However, he said he was feeling some improvement after following a suitable diet and taking vitamin B supplements.

When I examined him I found the typical results of a previous injury to his thoracic spine – intense spasm of the muscles from the neck to the lower thoracic part of the back.

These are by no means all the possible symptoms of the post-viral syndrome but Joe's is a good representative case. After treatment to his back, Joe's condition rapidly improved and he was soon back to full-time work.

## WHAT CAUSES POST-VIRAL SYNDROME?

This is the subject of much research, and the findings of different medical specialists, naturally enough, tend to lean towards their own particular area. Thus, a virologist – a bacteriologist who specializes in viral diseases – may believe it to be caused by a virus such as an entero virus, which mainly infects the bowel. Inevitably, there are those who believe it to be a psychological complaint, especially because the results of clinical tests are usually normal.

I believe it to be the result of an almost complete shutdown of the sympathetic nervous system. This is caused by two separate problems which, put together, give the picture of post-viral syndrome. The underlying problem is the wide-reaching effects of a severe injury to the chest area of the spine. As we have seen, such an injury can result in a low sympathetic drive, leading to chronic fatigue, with associated complaints. The second problem arises when a patient already suffering from a low sympathetic drive has an attack of influenza or similar acute infectious disease, which further upsets the sympathetic chain and lowers the body's resistance to infection.

## THE BODY'S OWN SEWAGE FARM

If a person has had an injury to the chest area of the spine as a result of, say, slipping and falling over backwards, there will be a protective spasm of the paravertebral muscles in this area. This will interfere with the normal function of the muscle pump and lead to a build-up of oedema both in the muscles themselves and also in the adjoining tissues. The sympathetic nerve centres may be affected by the build-up of oedema, leading to many of the symptoms of low sympathetic drive.

Unfortunately, the sympathetic nervous system is not the only system that may be involved. Intermingled with the ganglia are numerous *lymph nodes*. These are part of the lymphatic system, a special mechanism for dealing with an infection, damage or foreign bodies in the tissue spaces.

In order to get a good picture of the role of the lymph nodes it may help to look back to some of the points raised in chapter 1 concerning the circulation of the blood. We saw that when the blood reaches the capillaries, fluid diffuses from the blood into the tissue spaces taking in supplies and oxygen. It then diffuses back into the other end of the capillaries carrying with it carbon dioxide and waste products. The blood system is able to a great extent to keep out undesirable foreign bodies such as bacteria, viruses, white cells that have engulfed some invader, and the broken-down remains of debris.

During the transfer there is no direct connection between the blood vessels and the tissue spaces, so some mechanism for the removal and disposal of foreign bodies is needed. This is where the lymphatic system comes in (see figure 7.1). As the lymphatic ducts are in direct

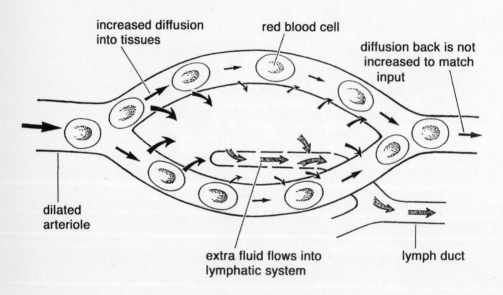

*Figure 7.1* When inflamed (by bruise or infection) the arteriole dilates, increasing the blood flow into the capillary, and thus into the tissue spaces. Some of this tissue fluid goes into the lymphatic system, taking with it bacteria, minute foreign bodies and white blood cells.

communication with the tissue spaces, they act as the sewers of the body and make it possible for these particles to be removed. The moment any infection gets into the tissue spaces, the bacteria, viruses and any foreign bodies are swept up into the lymph ducts by the tissue fluids, which are then called lymph. The driving force is a massive increase in the blood supply, which is part of the body's response to the infection, and of course the muscle pump.

The bacteria and viruses pass up the ducts either independently or after being engulfed in the white cell soldiers of the body. Either way, cells, other debris and undesirable chemicals present in the tissue spaces accompany them. After being processed to remove all these impurities, the lymph passes into the final lymph ducts and these join into the huge veins at the top of the chest. Lymph nodes filter and detoxify the lymph as it passes through.

As figure 7.2 shows, chains of lymph nodes ensure that the lymph is reasonably pure by the time it is returned to the bloodstream. This is important because the arterial system has little power to deal with such problems. At the same time, a special mechanism produces antibodies that are lethal to particular organisms. Each antibody works against one type of bacterium only, so the body has many antibodies to cover a wide range of bacteria and viruses.

Now, if the muscle pump is not working properly and there is a build-up of oedema in the local tissues, these lymph nodes, or filters, will also be affected. If they too are blown out with fluid, they may well become less efficient.

## SORE THROAT AND TONSILLITIS

If someone who already has a low sympathetic drive develops a sore throat or tonsillitis, this can easily lead to post-viral syndrome. Tonsils

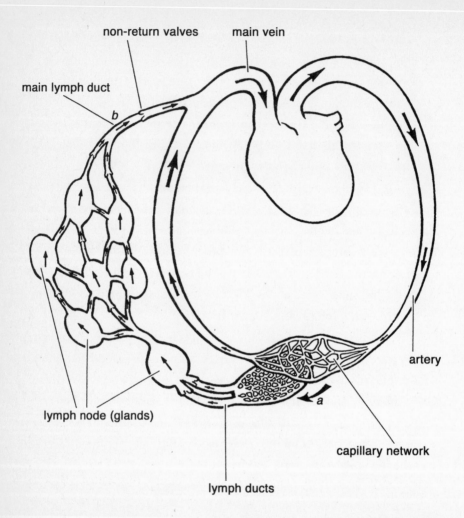

*Figure 7.2* The lymphatic system runs parallel to the circulatory system. At point *a*, the tissue fluids, containing waste, bacteria and minute solids, pass into the lymph, where they are cleaned. At point *b*, the main lymph duct, cleaned fluid and antibodies are returned to the vein, and the circulatory system.

produce antibodies to combat infections taken by mouth, but these antibodies may not be able to control a particularly virulent bacterium, in which case a sore throat and tonsillitis may result (see page 119).

Most of these bacteria, such as a haemolytic streptococcus, put out toxins to prevent the body from throwing them out. These inflame the throat membrane and pass into the blood stream inflaming any similar membrane in the body. Joint and muscle membranes are commonly the usual victims. With the tonsils largely destroyed, this state of affairs can go on for many, many years. In its lowered state of resistance, the body may not be able to combat any toxins that are released.

VIRAL INFECTION

If you go down with a viral infection, especially a fairly severe one such as flu, the lymphatic system has a great deal of work to do. If, as a result of a poor muscle pump action, the lymph nodes are already overloaded, they will become even more waterlogged than before. This, of course, makes it difficult to throw off the current infection and also lowers the body's resistance to any future infections. Thus, we have the usual history of an acute flu-like infection starting the illness off and then the seemingly never-ending milder recurrences of infection every few weeks or months.

Mary, a 21-year-old secretary, came to see me because she was feeling tired. She had been involved in a car crash when she was 18 and was sufficiently shaken and bruised to be taken to hospital for a check-up. Nothing major was found and she was discharged the same evening. The next day she saw her GP because she had a bad headache over her eyes and felt very stiff in her back. This settled down in the next few weeks but she never felt as well as she did before the accident.

One year later she went down with a viral infection that left her exhausted, but she got over this within a month. A few months later she had another viral attack, followed by flu-like attacks. These stopped after a couple of years. By now, however, she was so exhausted she had to give up work. A diet designed to avoid food intolerances helped but not enough to get her back to work.

She came to me with a list of symptoms including dizziness and indigestion, a woolly feeling in her head and a very poor memory. Examination revealed extensive spasm of the spinal muscles, especially in the thoracic region. Her blood pressure was low, she had a painful hip and shoulder joints, and her stomach was very tender. Her tonsils were large and infected and she had a number of large, tender lymph nodes in her neck.

Mary's tonsils were removed and I gave her physiotherapy and remobilization, and treated her lymph nodes with ultrasonic waves and massage for nearly three months. By this time she felt 80 per cent on the road to recovery. After another three to four months she went back to work feeling better than she could remember. The woolly feeling in her head was the last symptom to go, and was relieved by six magnesium injections.

## SYMPTOMS OF POST-VIRAL SYNDROME

### Complete exhaustion

A large number of lymph nodes are intermingled with the sympathetic nerve centres (see figure 7.3). As we have seen in chapter 6, these nerve centres control almost all the parameters of the body and are linked to the adrenalin mechanism. If someone is suffering from a low sympathetic drive, one of the main symptoms is fatigue. This is caused

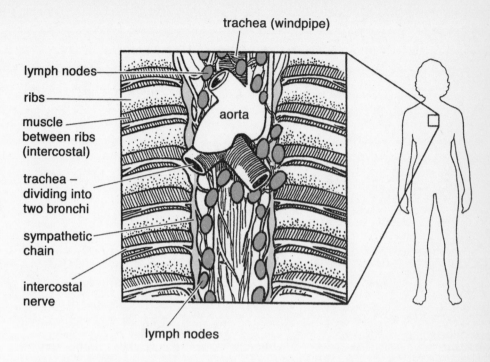

trachea (windpipe)

lymph nodes

ribs

muscle
between ribs
(intercostal)

aorta

trachea –
dividing into
two bronchi

sympathetic
chain

intercostal
nerve

lymph nodes

*Figure 7.3* The close proximity of the sympathetic nerve chain and the lymph nodes. Clearly, if the lymph nodes are inflamed, the nerve centres will become waterlogged.

by the poor action of the muscle pump, leading to a build-up of oedema in the tissue spaces, which chokes the sympathetic nerve centres and lowers their efficiency. If these nerve centres become even more waterlogged as a result of the inflammation of the adjacent lymph nodes, the feeling of tiredness will be even greater. In fact, it may be so great that you may be overwhelmed by exhaustion at the slightest effort.

There is another very important cause of the tiredness. Associated with the low sympathetic drive, or even caused by it, is a depressed output from the *pituitary gland*. The pituitary is a small ductless gland that lies at the base of the brain, just behind the nose, and secretes directly into the blood stream. One of its main purposes is to exercise overall control of the other ductless glands, including the adrenal, suprarenal cortex and thyroid glands. These produce noradrenaline, cortisol and thyroxin.

- **Noradrenaline** has a considerable effect on maintaining blood pressure and general energy levels. If it is insufficient, blood pressure is on the low side and you will tire easily.

---

LIQUORICE SWEETS

In Europe, a large number of substances are used to supplement the noradrenaline but they are not used in this country because of their side effects. Agitation and difficulty in sleeping are two common ones. A tendency to addiction is another. I have found that liquorice seems to put the blood pressure up a little, and appears to have no disadvantages. Two or three sweets a day are usually all that is necessary.

---

- **Cortisol** is a precursor of cortisone. It is difficult to replace for more than a few months as this will gradually lower the body's own output and eventually – usually after a period in excess of a year – can permanently suppress the body's own production. It is worth trying if allergies or food sensitivities are present because your own production usually increases before any major complication sets in. But if it does not suit you, as occasionally happens, it has to be abandoned.

■ **Thyroxin**, known as T3 for short, is one of five hormones secreted by the thyroid gland. It is not very active and is converted into T4, which is also secreted in small quantities by the thyroid, and which is very active. This is the substance that actually stimulates the metabolism of most tissues in the body. If the output is insufficient the person tires easily, tends to put on weight and the skin can be somewhat oily and become coarser. Thyroxin supplements add to the available natural output without affecting the body's production, so it can be administered for as long as it is needed. As many as 18 per cent of the population are estimated to be undiagnosed as short of thyroxin.

THYROXIN LEVELS

The blood test used to identify the degree of a thyroid problem is very inaccurate and cannot be relied on. Your doctor should give a small dose of thyroxin to start with and gradually increase it as needed until the optimum level is reached, leaving an interval of at least a week before changing doses. Too big a dose may result in occasional bouts of palpitations and/or agitation. The ideal is that you should feel well and be unaware of taking any supplements.

Some people do not respond very well to the thyroxin alone as their conversion to T4 is poor and they need a small dose of tertroxine (T4) to stimulate this. Rarely, even this is insufficient and the patient requires natural Armour thyroid, which contains a third substance called Gq/11 required to control the activity of the T4 in the cells.

Happily, thyroid production tends to improve as you recover, so the dose can often gradually be reduced and eventually discontinued.

Many people whose main symptom is complete exhaustion have a history of fibrositis between the shoulders and mild symptoms of a low sympathetic drive before the onset of severe illness.

Wendy, 38 and a keen sportswoman, came to me complaining of extreme fatigue. She had been a very energetic person for many years but she now felt permanently exhausted and could not understand why. As we talked, she revealed that she had suffered a bad attack of glandular fever six years previously. From then on she had never felt well. She suffered some indigestion, slept badly, felt very tensed up and had times of feeling depressed. She also had fibrositic pains between her shoulder blades. On examination, she had considerable spasm of the back muscles in the chest area, particularly between the shoulder blades. This is a typical picture of ME – especially as the clinical tests were normal. After eight treatments to her back she was fit and well again.

### Poor memory and a woolly feeling in the head

Tiredness and a woolly feeling are symptoms of magnesium deficiency in the red blood cells. This may come about as a result of poor absorption due to the stomach condition described below. Alternatively, stress or anxiety causes the body to excrete excessive amounts. People suffering the symptoms of ME and also having a poor memory, can be greatly helped by taking magnesium tablets. Occasionally, injections are needed if there is a poor response to tablets.

Indigestion, vitamin and mineral deficiencies, food allergy and candida infestation

■ **Indigestion.** One result of HST, or a low sympathetic drive, is indigestion. This is due to the excess acid in the stomach caused by parasympathetic over-activity. The excessive acid can inflame the stomach lining and impair the absorption of certain substances even though they may be plentiful in the diet. One of the first casualties of this is the vitamin B group. Shortage makes you feel even more tired and depressed.

■ **Vitamin and mineral deficiencies.** Whether for the same reason or not, patients suffering from post-viral syndrome often have a shortage of the trace elements zinc, magnesium and occasionally copper and chromium. These shortages can affect the function of the antibodies and so make it even more difficult to throw off an infection.

■ **Food allergy.** The inflammation of the stomach also makes it more sensitive, so certain substances that may irritate it a little can cause an allergic reaction (see page 108). You may respond with an acute reaction such as a strawberry rash, or there may be a more complex response. This is because the effect of the allergy itself is often over-ridden for an hour or two by a massive release of the body's natural cortisone, which is a powerful anti-allergen and gives a feeling of wellbeing. After the cortisone has worn off, you feel tired and depressed.

The sad thing is that the initial feeling of wellbeing makes those suffering from post-viral syndrome think that the particular food to which they are allergic is a saviour, and they resort to it frequently to try to regain fitness. This is exactly what happened to me.

Ten years ago I was thinking of retiring because I had been so tired for the previous year or so. I had a full check-up and nothing was found to be wrong. In fact, I was told that I was very fit. Undiagnosed tiredness is a common symptom in people coming to see me so I decided to give myself a consultation. Again, nothing seemed to be the cause until I thought of food intolerance. Suddenly, I realized my problem – coffee.

I had a cup of coffee before I got out of bed in the morning. The main attraction of breakfast was coffee. My secretary virtually faced the sack if I was not greeted with a cup, and at 11 I could not see another patient until I had consumed more. Lunch was highlighted by my post-prandial cup of coffee. An increase in consumption coincided to a large extent with the onset of my fatigue.

For this reason I became convinced that I was allergic to coffee. I stopped drinking it but within two days I knew that I could not continue working unless I had a cup. It was not until I went on holiday that I was able to give it up after two very difficult weeks.

In the case of a sensitivity, coffee stimulates a huge output of cortisone with an accompanying feeling of wellbeing. As the cortisone level drops below normal, this feeling changes to one of fatigue and depression, and another cup seems to be the way to get the feeling of wellbeing back. The lack of cortisone increases until the tiredness becomes overwhelming.

In my case, after many months one cup of coffee did not result in too excessive a drop in cortisone, so I was able to indulge myself occasionally.

There may be other symptoms of an allergy besides tiredness, such as aches between the shoulders; pain and swelling in some joints, perhaps the fingers or a knee; swollen ankles; abdominal disorders such as vague indigestion, bowel upsets and distension; headaches; catarrh; depression and even mental disorder. Skin and blood tests for allergies can give very good results.

---

### AN ELIMINATION DIET

If an allergic reaction is suspected, an elimination diet will help to identify the source. All substances known to cause an allergy are forbidden and then gradually re-introduced one at a time so that the culprit is discovered when the patient suffers a sharp reaction. Common offenders are dairy produce, white flour and coffee.

If you try a version of this for yourself, remember that it is important to eliminate more than one substance at a time. Either work out all the substances that could be causing the allergy and avoid eating them, or undertake a total elimination diet that excludes all known allergens. You will probably feel particularly bad at first. The improvement comes after about five days when the body has cleared itself of all the offending substances.

---

■ **Candida infestation.** Candida is a yeast-like fungus that is found virtually everywhere in the body. It is normally harmless to humans but may thrive in those who are rundown, suffering from a food allergy or vitamin B deficiency, eating a poor diet, often containing excessive sugar and, most important, taking antibiotics to fight infection. The colonies of helpful bacteria that compete with candida for space and food in the body are greatly diminished by the antibiotics so the candida can take over.

Candida produces a similar allergy to food but, unlike food, it is present all the time, so the cortisone becomes exhausted and permanent tiredness sets in. Candida is thought to be most active in the bowel where the irritation results in abdominal symptoms such as indigestion, distension and diarrhoea. Extensive testing, however, even snipping bits of the bowel out, have almost universally failed to demonstrate candida in the bowel except in the last days of the terminally ill. The obvious beneficial results of the usual anti-candida diet is now thought to be that the patient is sensitive to substances in the diet itself.

### Weakness of the joints

A number of people suffering from post-viral syndrome complain of weakness in a leg or an arm, and even that the limb suddenly gives way at times, causing them to stumble or drop things. Again, this could be due to the malfunction of the sympathetic nervous system. Low sympathetic drive can cause joints to become arthritic because normal repair does not restore them completely.

Many people complaining of weak limbs have an associated joint that is arthritic. When a joint is not in perfect working order, nature makes an attempt to give it a rest and increase its chance of healing by immobilizing it. Pain is the most obvious device, but it is also common for the nerve supply to the muscles working the joint to limit the power available. This gives the impression that the leg is heavy and not working very well, or that the arm or grip is weak. This weakness is not a neurological disorder but one of the normal mechanisms of repair. There is often a low level of pain in the limb at the same time, which may feel as if it comes from the muscles but almost certainly comes from the joint. The pain tends to decrease and finally vanish as the joint recovers.

An annoying extension of this is that, in moments of extra effort or stress, the nerves may cut off the muscle power almost completely for a brief second. This can cause the person to stumble or even fall, or to drop something they are holding. However, with correct diagnosis and treatment this can be helped.

When Margaret, 63, came to see me she said she had been suffering from arthritis for the past 15 years. Five years ago it had become very bad and she had had her toes operated on. She said she often woke with pain in her left shoulder and also had trouble in her left hip. The main problem, however, was her left hand. It was weak and painful all the time, especially in the cold weather. The first finger and wrist were the worst. She had recently dropped a plate of hot food when her wrist had given way. Margaret had been seeing an osteopath for 25 years for neck and back treatment. She had migraine attacks but no indigestion.

On examination, I found that her neck movements were below normal. Turning the head from side to side most easily assesses the normal movement of the neck – the chin should just about go over the shoulder and make an angle of 90 degrees. If the head will turn half this way only, to 45 degrees, the movement is said to be 50 per cent of normal. Margaret's head movements were 70 per cent normal.

There was an increase of the lumbar curve and the muscles were in considerable spasm. The sixth cervical and fourth lumbar vertebrae were tender. Various joints were swollen and tender, especially the left fingers and wrist. Tests for rheumatism were negative.

My diagnosis was that she had injured her back in the past, and that the oedema from the poor muscle pump had involved the sympathetic nerve centres. As a result of this, she had faulty repair of the various joints, causing the weakness and giving way of the wrist. This cleared up after 14 more visits, when her back was treated. She also had treatment to the various affected joints with ultrasonic waves and remobilization, and an anti-inflammatory drug to speed up the effect of the treatment. Although she still has slight pains at times, she sleeps well and feels stronger and better than she can ever remember.

## Depression

A common symptom of a low sympathetic drive, a viral infection and vitamin B and magnesium deficiencies, depression can also be in-built with some people. This is one of the effects of post-viral syndrome to need separate treatment because it can become severe and obstruct the whole recovery process, and it may not respond to my treatment alone. If a faulty fence at the top of a cliff results in an unfortunate person falling to the bottom, it may well not be sufficient to repair the fence. The victim may well require a bandage on a wound and a splint on a fracture.

In the medical sense, depression is a feeling of being unable to get going or start doing anything. It can be the most difficult effect of post-viral syndrome to treat. Fortunately, the majority of people who have been to see me respond very well to the treatment I offer to the back and lymph nodes.

It is probable that post-viral syndrome affects the level of serotonin, one of the brain's chemical messengers. A reduced quantity causes people to feel depressed and unwell. An antidepressant that slows the body's disposal of serotonin can effectively help sufferers, but it is important not to take the type that inhibits the uptake of noradrenaline. If you are already in a tense, agitated state as a result of the low sympathetic drive, pills that reduce the effect of noradrenaline can make you so tensed up that you will feel much worse.

## A POSITIVE APPROACH

What you can do to help yourself

■ **Try to keep as fit as possible.** It is very important to keep going. Graduated exercise can be of great help. The body weakens automatically the less you do, so it needs strengthening by exercise. Great care must be taken not to overdo it, especially in the early stages, so take the maximum possible without causing excessive fatigue – little and often is the motto.

■ **Modify your diet.** Coffee, dairy produce (and this means all dairy produce, including cheese, yoghurt and fromage frais as well as butter, milk and cream) and/or white flour can upset people. Sugar is often a cause of trouble and, if so, needs to be eliminated as completely as possible. Remember, it takes about five days to get the last traces of sugar and other foods out of the body, so just one lapse on the fourth day and you have to begin again. Think of the time gone as an investment not to be frittered away.

■ **Replace trace elements.** Vitamin B tablets or fluid (I think the synthetic type is the best), including vitamin B12 tablets, are better taken separately. Vitamins A, D and C help to increase resistance to infection – try taking vitamins A and D as cod or halibut liver oil in the recommended dosage, and up to 1 gram of vitamin C daily.

Among other elements often needed are iron, magnesium, manganese, chromium and zinc. These can be taken separately (zinc should always be taken on its own at night), or in a combined form with vitamin C.

Other remedies such as royal jelly may help but are of questionable value. General diet control may also be of assistance. Eat each group of foods separately – predominantly carbohydrates at one meal, protein at another. Some people find that avoiding red meat helps them.

■ **Massage the neck and back.** A friend or relative may be willing to help in this way. The massage should be firm and given for about 10 minutes. Massaging the lymph nodes in the neck often helps recovery from the infectious part of the illness.

■ **Contact a relevant association.** Various organizations offer support and advice about what your own doctor can do. The Useful Addresses section on page 290 has details of some of them.

■ **Consider replacing mercury fillings in your teeth.** This does dramatically help a few people but it is very expensive and in the majority of cases is of little help.

■ **Take a cold bath every morning.** A quick in and out of a cold bath gives the system a jolt and gets the noradrenaline mechanism on the move. Never do this without someone at hand to help you if something goes wrong.

Armed with the above advice, when you see your doctor, there are several things to ask about:

– treatment to the neck and thoracic spine as detailed in Appendix 1 'A note for your therapist' (page 249).
– having trace elements assessed. If low, red cell magnesium needs to be replenished by weekly intra-muscular injections. Ask also about the possibility of receiving intravenous or intra-muscular vitamin B two to three times a week. Note that the lower margin of normal is not adequate for most people suffering from post-viral syndrome, especially in the case of iron. The level should be at the top of the range.
– possible thyroid problems. Do everything you can to persuade your doctor to investigate your thyroid gland thoroughly, bearing in mind the unreliability of the blood test (see page 125).

If you feel just moderately improved by all these measures, you may require a course of Nystatin, which will last for at least two to three months. It is an anti fungal drug and really does help a number of post-viral sufferers for no known reason. The drug should be in pure form and not taken as a tablet. Powder is probably best, but capsules are available although rather expensive. The dose should be started fairly low and gradually increased as advised by your doctor.

Finally, general and moral support is of great help. It is demoralizing to feel ill and to have your life in tatters – and then to be told that there is nothing wrong. In my experience, the majority of post-viral syndrome sufferers can be helped to return to a full and rewarding life. Indeed, many say they haven't felt so fit and healthy for years.

# 9 TAKING YOUR BACK SERIOUSLY

## Your back as an unsuspected cause of other diseases

At the start of the siege of Madrid during the Spanish Civil War, General Mola said, 'I have four columns operating against Madrid and a fifth column inside.' In this chapter, we ask the question – is the spine a 'fifth column'?

Apart from the illnesses and conditions associated with the back that have already been mentioned, some specific complaints are, in my view, often caused by back problems but are seldom recognized as such. It cannot be overstated that treatment of the symptoms alone will do nothing to help the underlying trouble. If treatment is directed at the basic cause, a more effective and lasting relief can be obtained.

These individual complaints are determined by which ganglion, or group of nerve centres, is affected by the oedema, which is caused by muscle spasm due to a spinal injury (see page 10). In chapter 6, we discussed hyposympathetic tone syndrome (HST), in which a number of nerve centres are involved, giving rise to several symptoms. In themselves these symptoms are often fairly mild. However, when a single ganglion is affected, the symptoms are usually much more severe. For example, someone suffering from low sympathetic drive may have vague indigestion as one of the symptoms. When just one ganglion is involved, there is usually one dominant condition and it is correspondingly more pronounced, a gastric or duodenal ulcer for example.

The best way to consider the diseases brought about by back trouble is to look at what happens when the various ganglia are not functioning efficiently, starting at the top of the nerve chain and working downwards. Before continuing, however, it is important to understand fully my theory on the cause of back pain and related diseases. If you wish to refresh your memory, you should re-read chapter 4.

## STELLATE GANGLION

This lies at the base of the neck and has two main functions:

- to control the amount of blood that passes through the arteries to the head and arms
- to monitor the repair of tissues. In the context of this book, this applies particularly to the joints and tendons in the arm.

### MIGRAINE HEADACHES

When something goes wrong with the stellate ganglion's control of the flow of blood through the arteries to the head and arms, migraine headaches may result.

Arteries have circular muscles in their walls that can vary the internal diameter. Contracting these muscles reduces the diameter and, in smaller vessels, can close the artery completely. This facility enables the body to make a relatively small amount of circulating blood – about eight pints – supply a large area by an incredibly sophisticated form of irrigation. It has been estimated that with modern technology if we were to try to construct a human being, we would need at least 70 pints of blood to perform the same function.

Sensors detect when an area is short of supplies and full of waste products, and accordingly send impulses to the appropriate ganglia. These open up the vessels supplying the affected area until the situation is corrected. The nerve centres then close the supply to that area and open it up in another needy place. When the system is working efficiently, there is complete control of the amount of blood that goes to any one part of the body. Local controlling mechanisms also have an influence on the system.

If a ganglion's function is disrupted by surrounding oedema, and if it contains oedema itself, the circular muscles in the arterial walls may contract too fiercely, thereby narrowing the internal diameter abnormally, even shutting off smaller ones completely over a wide area.

### The cause of migraine headaches

If someone has suffered a previous injury involving the base of the neck – perhaps in a car accident or on the sports field – the stellate ganglion may be affected by the resulting oedema. Eventually, this group of nerve centres will reach a critical point as a result of poor drainage brought about by muscle spasm.

The actual trigger for a migraine is almost always pressure on the second cervical nerve root. This area, just below the skull about two inches from the centre, becomes very tender. The nerve may malfunction and stimulate the stellate ganglion to close off the circulation to the brain by causing a spasm of the internal carotid artery, so depriving the brain of oxygen and essential nutrients. The brain, however, cannot survive very long without oxygen so this arterial spasm is violently over-ridden, causing the artery to dilate over the area of its malfunction. The brain becomes flooded and as it is held within a rigid structure – the skull – this causes a considerable rise in pressure. The result of this is a migraine headache. Figure 8.1 shows some of the triggers of migraine on the stellate ganglion.

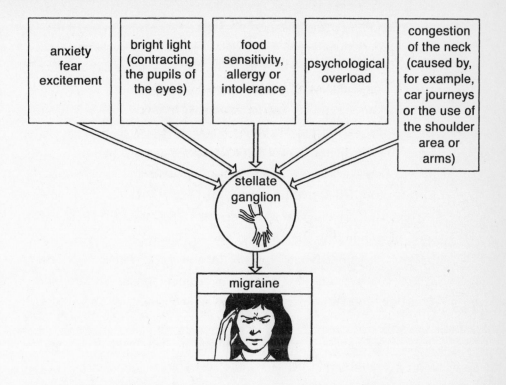

Figure 8.1 Some of the stimuli which trigger a migraine.

Lack of blood during the arterial spasm upsets the function of various nerve centres in the brain, which causes a number of corresponding symptoms, such as visual disturbance and pins-and-needles in, say, an arm or hand. Patients learn to recognize their own symptoms as indicating the onset of a headache.

The next stage, the flooding of the brain and increased pressure in the skull, causes headache, sickness, usually severe vomiting, and various other symptoms such as sensitivity to light and sound.

The arterial spasm is widely recognized as the cause of a migraine and the mainstay of treatment was to give drugs at the moment of onset containing ergotamine, which constricts the arteries to limit the flooding of the brain. Analgesics, such as aspirin, paracetamol or co-proxamol, may help to relieve the pain, and anti-sickness drugs, such as metoclopramide, can be taken as well to help control nausea and vomiting. An injection of a serotonin uptake inhibitor such as Imigran is very effective at stopping the headache at any stage of the attack. Drugs to prevent attacks have to be taken over a period of time. These include beta-blockers, such as propalalol, and serotonin antagonists, such as pitzotifen or rivotril.

None of these drugs cures the disease – they are merely different ways of minimizing the effect of the headaches. I believe that by treating the underlying problem in the back, rather than the symptoms, it is possible to give permanent relief. Richard and Christine, whose stories are told below, show the success of my theory.

Richard, a 56-year-old architect, told me he had begun suffering from migraine headaches at around five years of age. At first he didn't get them very often but they became more and more intense and frequent. By the time he was 10 he was having migraines every few days and had even begun to make himself sick as he found that this aborted the headache. Things had improved somewhat over the years but he still had severe migraine headaches fairly often. They were brought on by bright sunshine, becoming excessively tired, playing games or taking fairly heavy exercise, gardening and moderate or long motor journeys.

Richard tired very easily and had some fibrositis between his shoulders and at the base of his neck. On examination, his neck movement were about 70 per cent normal. There was intense spasm of the paravertebral muscles from the occiput, which is where the neck muscles join the skull, to the lower thoracic area. The muscles at the base of the skull were very tender. After seven visits, when his neck and upper thoracic spine were treated, Richard still had slight headaches but no migraine. He left feeling on top of the world. However, the migraines returned a year later following a stressful period of his life. He had three more treatments and has had no further trouble since then.

Like many migraine sufferers, Christine, a 34-year-old mother of three, has to stay in a dark room when she has an attack because she feels sick and is upset by the slightest sound or light.

Christine came to me because she had been suffering from severe headaches for nearly 20 years. On two occasions a cluster of these headaches had become so severe she was hospitalized. She had been given many drugs and diets but, with the exception of ergotamine tablets, none of these had really helped. She tired very easily, had dizzy spells, indigestion, low blood pressure and generally felt washed out.

When I examined Christine, I found an extreme tenderness just under the skull. The muscles were so tight or hard in spasm that the extra pressure from my fingers was enough to produce pain. Her neck movements were 70 per cent normal. Over seven visits her neck and thoracic spine were treated to relieve the neck problem, which then improved the muscle pump. As the oedema began to reduce, the headaches began to subside. After three to four months, they gave her no further trouble.

If you are a migraine sufferer you will sympathize with Richard and Christine. You too may have been searching for many years for some clues to why you suffer attacks and what you can do to prevent them.

If the stellate ganglion is indeed the usual cause of migraine headaches, the theory will provide answers to many of your questions and explain why certain factors are likely to precipitate a crisis. The most common times to get a migraine are

- when you wake up in the morning
- when you are tired, anxious or excited
- in bright light, especially in spring sunshine
- after eating certain foods including chocolate
- after car journeys
- after exercise of the shoulder girdle, such as when using a computer keyboard or playing tennis

*Why is it that after a night's rest I wake up with a migraine ?*

During the night there is little or no movement to activate the muscle pump adequately. The body becomes marginally congested, although the milking effect of the vein walls and the pumping effect of breathing keeps this at an acceptable level. If, however, there is muscle spasm in the cervical and upper thoracic muscles, there will already be excessive fluid in the surrounding tissues. During the night the increase in this fluid can be enough to upset the stellate ganglion and result in a migraine. This is a common trigger of a headache.

*Why is it that as soon as I get excited I have a migraine attack?*

Anything that stimulates the stellate ganglion, or the whole sympathetic system, is a possible trigger. We have already seen that fear, tension and anxiety stimulate the sympathetic system to prepare you to cope efficiently in an emergency (see page 102). Thus these emotions are often found to be the cause of a migraine, and excitement can be added to the list.

Under primitive conditions, excitement did not exist in the way we know it today. There was no such thing as excitement at the prospect of some happy occasion, such as going out on a special date. It is only since humans have developed the power of speech and communication that we can look forward to events. This being so, excitement is muddled with fear by the subconscious and both produce adrenalin. As far as the stellate ganglion is concerned, a person reacts in the same way whether they are excited at the thought of a forthcoming party or terrified as they face a mugger with a sharp knife.

Excitement is a common cause of migraine. Many sufferers get an attack just before they are about to go on holiday or when they are about to do something they have been looking forward to for some while.

*Why do I so often get a migraine on a sunny day?*

The pupil of the eye is to some extent controlled by the stellate ganglion, which allows it to contract with the stimulation of bright light. So when the weather suddenly becomes sunny with bright clear skies – especially at the beginning of spring – this can trigger off attacks. It is not clear why the April sun causes migraine reactions. It is possible that after winter, the bright sunshine may be more difficult to adjust to than later when the brain becomes more used to the light.

*Why do some foods cause migraine headaches?*

When you eat food that is difficult to digest or to which you are allergic, the stomach needs an extra supply of blood to help it cope.

Blood is diverted to the stomach from other areas. If the stellate ganglion is malfunctioning, instead of a mild contraction diminishing the blood supply to the brain, a spasm takes place, cutting it off altogether, and that precipitates a headache.

Unfortunately, the same condition that makes you prone to migraines also makes you susceptible to food sensitivities. This is because the nerve centre that controls acid to the stomach is near the stellate ganglion and so is often involved to some extent in the waterlogging. As a result, there may be an excess of acid in the stomach, which can make it at least slightly inflamed. This produces conditions whereby sensitivities and later allergies to food can readily come about.

Such food sensitivities can be a common cause of triggering a headache, but they are only one of the possible causes. Fortunately, if the excess acid disappears, as the conditions causing the migraine are treated, the sensitivity to the food will often settle down and thus not cause any more headaches. It is, however, sometimes necessary to take active steps to deal with the food allergy.

*Why do migraines often start after a long car journey?*

On a car journey your neck has to do a lot of work keeping your very heavy head upright during braking, accelerating and cornering. To cope with the extra effort, your neck muscles need a considerably increased supply of blood but, as there is very little actual movement of the head, the muscle pump is relatively ineffective. This results in a build-up of oedema in the base of the neck, which upsets the stellate ganglion and causes the onset of a headache.

*Why is it that a migraine starts several hours after chopping wood?*

Extra activity with the arms – such as chopping wood, playing some games or lifting weights – increases the muscular activity in the shoulders and neck and likewise increases the arterial supply. During the actual work, the muscle pump is quite effective and the tissue fluids remain at a reasonable pressure. Unfortunately, the greatly increased supply of blood to the muscles does not immediately die back once the work is completed but fades away over a period of time. While the blood supply is still excessive, it floods the neck area after you have stopped the activity and this may trigger a migraine even some hours later.

*Is it true that migraine is a psychological disease?*

A number of people believe that migraine is a psychological disorder. It is my belief that migraine is purely physical, brought about by the causes described above. However, it is not unusual to have a psychological overlay superimposed on a physical condition. This is a rather long-winded way of saying that conditioned reflexes develop. Think of a dog at feeding time. If you ring a bell and then feed the dog, he will associate the food with the bell and come whenever you ring it. If, after a long period of time, you stop feeding the dog but continue to ring the bell, the dog will react as follows. First he will come whenever you ring it but after a while he will become more reluctant and then not come at all.

In humans, the subconscious can note that a headache prevents you from doing something you find unpleasant, such as visiting an unpopular aunt or going to school when you have not done your homework. So when a similar occasion arises, your subconscious may mimic a headache – which you believe to be a genuine migraine – as an escape mechanism. In some people, the induced headaches can outnumber the genuine attacks.

Fortunately, if the physical cause can be disposed of – as when you stop feeding the dog – the psychological attacks gradually fade out and cease to be a problem.

---

CERVICAL TENSIONAL HEADACHE

A headache very similar to migraine results when the external instead of the internal carotid artery is affected, but without the preliminary signs or the nausea and vomiting. The headache can be very severe and often seems to start in one temple or the other. It is more common than migraine and brought on by a similar set of conditions, so the two are often confused. A cervical tensional headache usually radiates towards the back of the head and may reach as far as the root of the neck. I believe the pain to be caused by the walls of the artery going into a cramp and this can be crippling.

---

ARTHRITIS OF THE SHOULDER AND HAND

Any trouble in a joint is called arthritis – from 'arthros' meaning joint and 'itis' meaning inflammation. The stellate ganglion monitors the repair of tissues in the joints and tendons of the arm, and the repair mechanism is normally very efficient. People who complain of painful joints are often told that it is because the joints are wearing out – 'What do you expect at your age?' What age? I see a number of people under the age of 20 with joint pains, very many in middle age and probably a similar number of older people. At what point are they wearing out?

Based on my experience, I do not believe that under normal circumstances we actually wear out during our lifetime.

If you bought a very fine car and ran it 12 or more hours a day every day of the year, the bearings would probably be worn after, say, five years. One would assume that the joints in the body are moderately superior to a car's bearings, so they may be expected to show marked wear after 10 or 15 years. The fact that this does not happen is because each time a joint becomes worn, sensors in it send impulses to the appropriate sympathetic ganglion, which initiate the multiplication of cells until, helped by local reactions, all wear has been restored. This repair system slows down with age, but so does your level of activity to match it. I believe that if a joint is suffering from wear, it is because something, somewhere, has gone wrong with the repair mechanism.

Emily first felt discomfort in her left knee when she was 66 years old, 12 years before coming to see me. The discomfort occurred randomly and as it had not stopped her getting around she didn't seek medical advice. But around her 73rd birthday, the pain started in her other knee as well and this became much worse, beginning to make walking difficult. A consultant told her that it was arthritis because of her age and an operation to replace the knee might be needed if it became very bad. Physiotherapy helped a little, but the pain in the knee slowly became more obtrusive.

She told me she had suffered from mild lumbago on and off for 20 years. On examination, I found her two knees were swollen and painful with limited movement. Her back had almost no lumbar curve and there was a considerable amount of spasm of the muscles caused by an old injury that had bruised the facet joints.

After 11 visits, during which time her lumbar spine was treated to improve the facet joints, the spasm was gradually resolved. At the same time, she was given treatment to her knee with traction, massage and ultrasonic waves to accelerate the repair. As this happened, she began to feel much better and her knees began to improve as the function of the lumbar sympathetic ganglion was restored. She had three more visits over the next three months, by which time the knees were no longer swollen. However, she still feels some discomfort in her right knee when going upstairs. Unfortunately, I can suggest no reason for this.

Once the repair mechanism can be made to work effectively again, the joint will be restored to good order, whatever the person's age, as the success of the treatment to Emily's knee shows.

Treating the joint as well as the underlying back problem greatly accelerates recovery. If the shoulder is the problem, I use ultrasonic waves, massage, manipulation and exercises. Freezing the joint reduces excessive circulation, which can help speed up recovery. I find that frozen peas are one of the best mediums for this, applied direct to the shoulder for one and a half minutes every day.

There may come a time, however, when you cannot recover with this treatment. A normal joint has very smooth surfaces of cartilage and a special fluid oils the joint and reduces the friction (and therefore wear) to a very low level. As the cartilage wears and becomes slightly rough, it acts as fine sandpaper on the other side of the joint and so the wear in the joint increases considerably with each movement. Eventually, a stage is reached where the ability to replace cells is exceeded by the destruction of them and then it is no longer possible for the joint to recover. Fortunately, this occurs only after a great deal of wear has taken place.

Emergency action

If the stellate ganglion is not functioning properly, the repair of the joint is inadequate. There may be no initial symptoms but over a period of time the wear becomes significant and, eventually, it may become critical, or you may do something unusual or undertake an activity that involves the joint in extra exertion. In either case, the stellate ganglion is made aware that it is a year or so behind with its repair mechanism and is prompted into action.

Instead of gently speeding up repair as it would normally do, the stellate ganglion panics and rings the alarm bells. An emergency repair mechanism is immediately put to work, which produces an inflammatory reaction whereby the blood supply is greatly increased to the affected tissues in the shoulder and hands. The extra oxygen and nutrients from this new supply of blood make the joints considerably better for a short time but the relief is temporary. The emergency reaction also creates a sensation of pain, making you aware of the joints in order to prevent use of them. This increased awareness of the shoulder or hand creates painful sensations under conditions that would not have caused any trouble before the first attack.

To illustrate this point, compare the stellate ganglion to a farm manager in charge of the day-to-day running of a large farm. If you are a prosperous farm owner you may well employ a manager to look after the ordinary running, repair and maintenance of the farm without necessarily referring back to you. The stellate ganglion is the manager of the upper part of the body and it will perform these functions without there being any conscious awareness of the things needing to be done or even the fact that they are being repaired.

If a neighbour telephones you to complain that his prize dahlias have been trampled by your cows, the chances are you would make an irate phone call to your manager to ask what is going on. He will explain that a short length of fence has fallen down allowing the cows to escape. You may well be extremely annoyed by this inefficiency and insist on being informed if so much as a stick comes out of any fence in future. So, after this incident, the manager will inform you of trivial matters that would previously have been dealt with without consultation.

In the same way, once the body had been made aware of the shoulder and hand, it reacts to even the most minor change in conditions. Just as the manager telephones the owner of the farm, so the conscious brain is made aware of each episode by messages producing the sensation of pain.

Alexander, a 47-year-old teacher, came to me complaining of rheumatoid arthritis. His fingers and wrists were swollen and painful and other joints, particularly his shoulders, had become fleetingly troublesome but had improved on their own. Blood tests were all negative.

On examination, I found considerable spasm of the paravertebral muscles throughout his back. When I asked about any previous injuries, he remembered that he'd had a bad fall from a horse 21 years before and had been suffering from slight backache fairly frequently for about six years. He had been to an osteopath on a number of occasions, both for backache and for pain in his left shoulder. He said he had been feeling tired and unwell for around six years.

The fall had damaged his paravertebral joints and the steady build-up of oedema in his back tissues had become bad enough for him to have a drop in his sympathetic drive six years earlier. This caused the fatigue that had started at that time. Even in those periods when extra activity had reduced the oedema enough to eliminate the pain, the problem in the back remained the same, and the brain continued to be conscious of the tiredness. As well as the tiredness, the low sympathetic drive also caused the problem in the fingers, which remained constantly painful. When he first felt pain, he remembers his fingers being quite swollen around the joints.

After seven visits, the spasm in Alexander's back was relieved to a great extent. The fingers were about 70 per cent better and he said he was feeling much improved in himself. Three months later his fingers had almost recovered but still felt painful the day after he had used them a great deal. Six months later all the pain had gone and Alexander said he couldn't believe how well he felt.

If the stellate ganglion is not working efficiently, the fingers can be very painful. This is because they are in constant use. If the normal repair mechanism is not functioning properly, the build-up of wear over the years will reach a critical point and the alarm bells will start ringing. The emergency repair mechanism is set in motion, which causes an abnormal reaction of swelling and pain. As time passes, the fingers can become increasingly painful, especially if the hands are used a great deal.

Charlotte, 61, was at her wits' end when she came to see me. Three years before she had been mugged and when her attackers snatched her handbag she clung on so tight that the first finger of her right hand was dislocated. She said she had suffered pain from the finger right up to the elbow ever since and this could be very bad at times. Her hand was very weak and did not seem to respond to any treatment.

She mentioned that she had been involved in a car crash 15 years before and had suffered a fairly severe whiplash injury. Her neck had been stiff on and off ever since. She was also suffering from high blood pressure.

She could not straighten the first finger of her right hand. The knuckles were very tender and her hand was so weak she could not make a fist. Her neck movements were restricted and there was considerable swelling at the base. Tension resulting from this unpleasant episode may well have further tightened the neck and shoulder muscles in the 'fight' reaction (see page 102), and further aggravated the condition.

On palpation, I found there was a spasm of the paravertebral muscles from the skull to the mid-thoracic region and the sixth cervical vertebra was very tender. Although the long-standing neck trouble had been reasonably stable for some time, it had flared up after the mugging, which had also damaged the joints in her hand. The hand was not repairing itself owing to defective monitoring of repair as the oedema around the stellate ganglion had interfered with its function. The stellate ganglion responded well to treatment of the neck area and when I saw her a year later for another problem, she said the hand had remained symptom-free.

As this case shows, treatment of the neck area will usually produce a marked and fairly rapid improvement in shoulder and hand problems, even to the point of complete relief, in most people. Curiously, shoulder problems usually occur in people in their twenties to forties and fingers start to give trouble thereafter.

## FROZEN SHOULDER

Inflammation caused by the malfunctioning of the stellate ganglion results in the shoulder becoming very painful and throbbing. In some cases, movement is reduced to almost nothing. Once the original crisis in the nerve centre is over, the trouble usually repairs itself and the shoulder gets better. Treatment to the stellate ganglion can speed up recovery time to weeks rather than months or a year.

The shoulder itself should also be treated with ultrasonic waves and exercises.


## TENNIS ELBOW

This condition got its name because a backhand tennis shot puts considerable strain on the muscle of the forearm at the place where it is fixed to the bone, just above the elbow on the thumb side, and excess strain here often causes the problem. The muscle runs down the forearm and attaches at the other end just above the wrist. If there is even a slight weakness in the maintenance system, this muscle is vulnerable to damage.

Muscles may be attached to a bone over a wide area, or by a single tendon. Tendons, which are like hard wires, form where a bulk of muscle would interfere with the freedom of movement of a joint, or where the muscle is situated a distance away from the second place of attachment. For example, the muscles in the forearm go into a long tendon that moves the fingers – fingers are too small to have the necessary sized muscles attached.

The forearm muscle is attached over a wide area and if some of the fibres become detached, acute pain at the elbow results whenever the wrist is turned – the damaged muscle has to contract in order to turn the wrist.

Many activities other than playing tennis can, of course, bring about the same injury. It is a persistent condition and tends to recur even if it is put right with injections of cortisone or other treatment. The simplest way to offer permanent relief is to treat the errant stellate ganglion.

John, 53, an enthusiastic sportsman, had started to have bad tennis elbow about six years before he came for a consultation. At the time, he had been given a cortisone injection with immediate, complete relief. Three years later, the pain started again and he had further injections. This time there was some relief and he was able to resume playing tennis. However, in the past 18 months the trouble had become very severe, and he got no relief from cortisone.

He told me that his neck had been mildly troublesome following a skiing accident 12 years before but it had never required any treatment. He also had very mild indigestion at times.

On examination, I could feel a small knot just above the right elbow, which was accompanied by the typical very tender area. His neck movements were almost normal but there was considerable spasm of the muscles from below the skull to the middle of the thoracic area. It was this that was causing oedema in the region of the stellate ganglion, causing his indigestion and delaying the healing of the tear in the muscle at the elbow.

John had seven sessions of treatment to his neck, and as this improved, so slowly did the elbow. A year later, it became uncomfortable again and three more visits were needed but since then the problem has not recurred.

A very similar condition is known as golfer's elbow. In this instance, another muscle is torn at the point where it is fixed to the bone just above the elbow, but on the other side. This is also caused by problems at the base of the neck and can be treated in the same way as tennis elbow. I have not seen a single case of tennis or golfer's elbow without accompanying neck, and therefore back, trouble.

Clifford had had bad tennis elbow 12 years before his first visit to me. An injection of cortisone had completely stopped the pain until four years later when a backhand at tennis caused the trouble to recur. He had another two injections of cortisone, which made it feel better but not completely right. Later still, he had physiotherapy with little improvement. A visit to an osteopath made the elbow feel better but it kept relapsing.

When I saw Clifford, he volunteered that he had had neck trouble since being in a motor car that was hit in the back, jerking his neck. The accident had taken place eight years before his first pain in the elbow.

After 11 treatments to his neck, Clifford's elbow was about 75 per cent better. In the following 12 weeks the pain disappeared completely. Two years later he had a twinge of pain and came to see me again. His neck muscle spasm had returned slightly. Three more visits got rid of this and he has had no further pain.

## CARPAL TUNNEL SYNDROME

The pain caused by this condition is felt mostly below the wrist, but it can radiate up the arm towards the elbow. Symptoms include numbness or pins and needles in the thumb, first finger and the nearside of the middle finger. There can be weakness of the thumb. A thickening of the ligament that strengthens the wrist on its palm side causes the problem. This runs in a thick band from one side of the wrist to the other. The median nerve that supplies the thumb and fingers with both sensation and muscle control passes through a tunnel in the ligament, known as the carpal tunnel.

If the stellate ganglion is not working at its best, this large ligament may not be properly maintained. In an attempt to give itself the extra strength needed, the ligament begins to thicken. This can result in the median nerve to the thumb, first finger and half the middle finger becoming pinched as it goes through the carpal tunnel. It is the pinched nerve that gives rise to the symptoms (see figure 8.2).

If the condition is not too bad, improving the circulation around the stellate ganglion can treat it. If, however, it is very severe or long established, it may be necessary to operate. Slitting the ligament along the line of the carpal tunnel and thus freeing the nerve from the pinching effect is a very simple, effective cure.

## RAYNAUD'S DISEASE

Vascular problems may also be associated with the stellate ganglion and one of the most common is Raynaud's disease in which the arteries taking supplies and oxygen to the tissues in one or both hands go into spasm and the hand becomes white and numb. The disease, which can be painful, is usually triggered by cold, for instance putting your hand in cold water. In lesser versions, people find that their hands, or just one hand, feel particularly cold. Much more rarely, it works the other way and the hand is permanently hot.

Raynaud's disease is difficult to treat. As the stellate ganglion directly controls the internal diameter of the artery in the arms, it follows that malfunction of the ganglion can cause spasms of the artery as a faulty response to cold, when you would normally expect it to close the artery slightly to conserve heat.

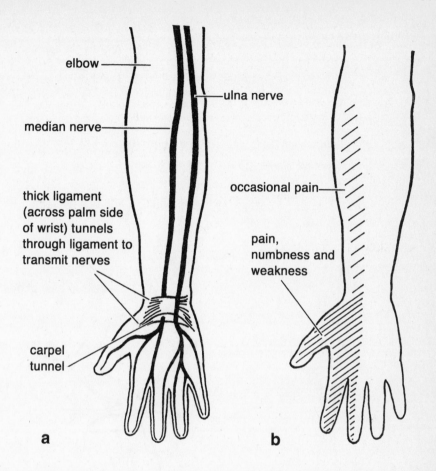

elbow

ulna nerve

median nerve

thick ligament
(across palm side
of wrist) tunnels
through ligament to
transmit nerves

occasional pain

pain,
numbness and
weakness

carpel
tunnel

a

b

*Figure 8.2* Carpal Tunnel Syndrome. Diagram *a* shows the thickening ligament, on the thumb side, pinching the nerve, causing pain and numbness. Diagram *b* shows the distribution of pain and numbness.

Successful treatment of the stellate ganglion does not always work as well as might be expected. The recognized treatment is to remove the stellate ganglion completely. However, since the sympathetic chain tends to reform, the disease returns.

## SPLANCHNIC GANGLION

This group of nerve centres lies in the middle of the thoracic spine (see figure 8.3). The two main functions are:

- to control the amount of acid in, and movements of, the stomach
- to control the blood supply to the abdomen

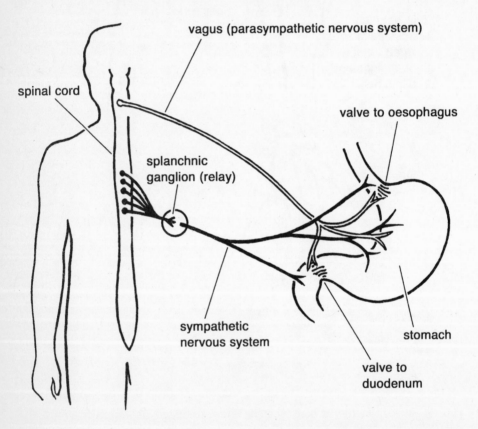

Figure 8.3 The nerve supply to the stomach. The parasympathetic nervous system initiates all digestive processes, following digestion from start to finish. The sympathetic nervous system turns off the stomach when no food is present – or when the body is experiencing fright or stress.

INDIGESTION AND FLATULENCE

Indigestion is "the inability to put a square meal into a round stomach" and it may signal that something is going wrong with the splanchnic ganglion. To be strictly accurate, the splanchnic ganglion opposes the vagus nerve, which is part of the parasympathetic nervous system. The vagus controls the digestive system (see chapter 6).

When food is swallowed it passes down the oesophagus into the stomach. At the entrance to the stomach, a ring of powerful muscles – a sphincter, as it is called – relaxes to allow the food to enter and then contracts to prevent the food and acid returning into the oesophagus. The food has to stay in the stomach until that part of the digestive process is complete. Its progress to the small intestine – the duodenum – is blocked by another sphincter, or valve. At the right moment, this relaxes to allow the stomach content to flow into the duodenum.

The vagus nerve is in a state of balance with the sympathetic nervous system. Each puts out a 'voltage' that under neutral conditions cancels the other out and maintains a healthy harmony. If, however, you have back trouble in the middle of the thoracic spine – and remember, you may not be aware of this – this will cause a partial failure of the muscle pump, leading to a build-up of oedema in the affected area. This may well depress the activity of the splanchnic ganglion, causing it to malfunction.

Upsetting the balance

This malfunction of the splanchnic ganglion causes an excess of acid in the stomach. Under resting conditions, if a person is not eating anything and is in a tranquil state, little acid is produced in the stomach. If, however, the parasympathetic pull is less opposed by the diminished sympathetic drive, the balance shifts in its favour and excessive acid is produced in the stomach even when there is no food present.

As I explained earlier (page 102), it helps to picture the vagus nerve and sympathetic nervous system as two teams in an equal tug-of-war contest. If one member of a team is removed, his team are no longer a match for the other and the rope will be pulled relentlessly across the line. In the case of the stomach, lowering sympathetic activity results in acid and digestive juices continuing to be secreted even after food has been fully digested. Also, the stomach carries on churning and the sphincters to the oesophagus and the duodenum possibly become a little slack. Figure 8.3 illustrates the close relationship between the vagus nerve and the digestive system.

In the early stages of imbalance, this results in mild indigestion. The most common symptom is that you nibble all day in a subconscious attempt to mop up the acid in the stomach.

In a more advanced condition, the inflammation of the stomach wall caused by the extra acid results in loss of appetite. This is the body's way of trying to rest the inflamed system. What seems like flatulence is also a common symptom at this stage as the patient swallows air in a subconscious attempt to keep the inflamed membranes apart and so stop them sticking together and irritating each other.

Treatment to the back in the area of the splanchnic ganglion will almost always clear up any indigestion and flatulence by restoring the balance with the parasympathetic nervous system.

## GASTRIC AND DUODENAL ULCERS

The next stage on from indigestion and flatulence depends on several factors:

- whether or not you have a built-in weakness in your digestive system that may be congenital
- the relative amount of movement versus acid in your stomach. In some people, the stomach churns forcefully and tends to push the acid into the duodenum; in others, the movement is more tranquil leaving the acid to burn a hole in the stomach wall
- lifestyle, especially eating habits. Irregular eating puts stress on the stomach because acid may form in expectation of a meal that doesn't arrive. Bus drivers used to be notorious for irregular eating and for having stomach-ulcer problems.

A *gastric ulcer* results when mild stomach contractions allow the acids to remain in the stomach where they will eventually burn a hole in the lining. A duodenal ulcer arises when the stomach contractions are stronger and the acid is squeezed through the sphincter into the duodenum. This normally contains alkaline juices, so it is not used to coping with acids and a hole is burned in its lining.

Tension is often blamed as a major contributor to a gastric or duodenal ulcer. My contention is that this tensed-up state is actually part of the same problem that causes the ulcer. Let me explain my reasoning.

You will by now be familiar with the effects of a low sympathetic drive, as discussed previously. One of the body's reactions is to try to increase the drive through a compensatory mechanism in the brain, which stimulates the anxiety/fright centre. As a result, you feel anxious and tensed up. It is probable that the state of anxiety stimulates the sympathetic/adrenalin system and thus helps to switch off the secretion of acid and the movements of the stomach, and so may in fact help reduce the cause of the inflammation of the stomach.

Tranquillizers are often helpful in the treatment of ulcers because they cause a relaxation of the muscle spasm in the back and this diminishes the low sympathetic drive.

Both gastric and duodenal ulcers can usually be cured successfully by treatment to the lower neck and the upper half of the thoracic spine, which corrects the malfunction of the splanchnic ganglion.

---

## GO TO THE DOCTOR!

If the indigestion is severe or an ulcer has been diagnosed, these should be investigated and treated in an orthodox manner at the same time as the back is being treated. Serious complications could occur before the back treatment has effected any major improvement.

---

## HIATUS HERNIA

This is another condition greatly aggravated by the malfunction of the splanchnic ganglion. The most obvious symptom is a burning sensation under the breastbone, which is particularly noticeable at night or whenever you lie down. The symptoms of simple indigestion are often attributed to a hiatus hernia if one is found, when the stomach is X-rayed. However, indigestion is seldom caused by a hiatus hernia.

As figure 8.4 shows, the diaphragm divides near the backbone to allow the big arteries and veins, the oesophagus and other structures to pass from the chest into the abdomen and vice versa. If the diaphragm has a larger hole than is necessary for this purpose, some of the stomach may well pass through the gap into the chest cavity, dividing itself into two parts shaped rather like an hourglass. This is a hiatus hernia. Obviously, the normal function of the stomach is interfered

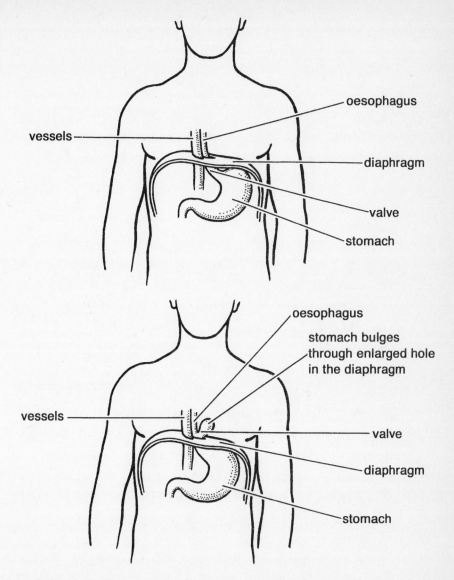

*Figure 8.4* Diagram *a* shows a normal oesophagus, passing through the close-fitting hole in the diaphragm. Diagram *b* shows a hiatus hernia, where the valve has become stretched, and food and acid regurgitate into the oesophagus – inflaming it and causing a burning pain under the lower part of the breast bone.

with. In particular, it can causes acid to pass up into the oesophagus when you are lying down, hence the discomfort at night.

Treatment to the area of the splanchnic ganglion will tighten the sphincter where the oesophagus goes into the stomach and may go a long way to relieving the symptoms of regurgitation caused by the hiatus hernia. It will, of course, also lessen the resting acid levels and thus help to relieve any indigestion that may be present.

ABDOMINAL MIGRAINE

The second function of the splanchnic ganglion is to control the supply of blood to the abdomen. If the nerve centres are not functioning as they should be, this can cause the artery to the intestines to go into cramp, causing a severe abdominal pain, usually accompanied by nausea and a feeling of general ill health. This is an abdominal migraine. It almost always responds well to treatment to the mid-thoracic area.

Mary, 34, told me her first attack had occurred just over three years previously, and had begun about an hour after lunch. She had suffered severe cramp-like pain in a wide area of the abdomen and had felt unwell and nauseous.

The next attack, around two years later, was similar. She suffered two more attacks during the next year. They all began around half an hour to two hours after eating and there was no obvious reason for them. She had been fully investigated for an abdominal problem in hospital but everything appeared to be normal.

Mary said she had been feeling rather low and had been tiring easily for several years. She had mild indigestion at times and a very occasional, slight ache between the shoulders.

On examination of the stomach, I found nothing abnormal. The back, however, showed considerable spasm of the paravertebral muscles in the mid-chest region. Her blood pressure was on the lowest level of normal. I diagnosed abdominal migraine and treated her thoracic spine. After eight visits she has remained free from attacks for 10 years.

## RELIEF FROM DEPRESSION AND OTHER TROUBLES

Patients like Mary who suffer from abdominal migraine and other complaints associated with the malfunction of the splanchnic ganglion are often amazed at their rapid recovery after treatment to the affected area in the back, namely the lower neck and upper half of the thoracic spine. Not only is there a marked improvement in their symptoms but also they feel altogether more energetic and better generally. They also lose the feeling of anxiety and tension which is often present.

It is very common for people with back trouble in this area to suffer depression. This is because when the activity of the anxiety centre – stimulated to galvanize the adrenalin mechanism when it is suffering from a low output – goes beyond an acceptable level, the brain tries to resolve the problem with the sensation of depression.

As with all the ganglia in the body, one or more things may go wrong, with mild or serious consequences. This will depend on a number of factors, including which part of the body is under greatest strain, what has been injured, or infected, or be subject to an inherited weakness. Most people do suffer to some extent or other. When I feel oedema around the splanchnic ganglion, I ask the patient if he or she tires easily, has indigestion or suffers from dysmenorrhoea (heavy and painful periods). The answer is usually yes to one or all of these.

After treatment, patients feel much more relaxed and freer in the shoulder and spine. Indeed, as one patient said to me, 'I had not realized my back had caused so many other problems. I would put up with my painful back so long as I could continue feeling so much better generally.' Many others say the same kind of thing. Fortunately, the back pain is usually expunged as well.

## LUMBAR SYMPATHETIC GANGLION

This group of nerve centres lies in the mid to upper lumbar region of the spine. Its functions are local, so the patient's general health is not involved and there are no symptoms of tiredness or anxiety when the nerve centres do not work as they should. The lumbar ganglion's functions are:

- to control the flow of blood through the arteries of the lower part of the body
- to control repair and maintenance in this part of the body

The two areas most affected by a breakdown are the hip and knee joints. For some curious reason, painful knees seem to be a feature of people from 10 to 30, while older people tend to suffer more from pain and eventually arthritis in the hip joint.

### ARTHRITIS OF THE HIP JOINT

The common arthritis covered by this book occurs when the repair mechanism of the joint becomes defective and cannot keep pace with wear, resulting in the slow deterioration of the joint. An ailing joint endeavours to buttress itself by increasing the bearing surface, so irregular bone begins to form around the edges. If the repair mechanism can be restored to normal or near it, it will start to outpace the wear again and the joint will make a significant recovery.

'Please do something about my hip,' pleaded 51-year-old Alice, who had been in considerable pain for two years. Her left hip was so uncomfortable she found it difficult going up and down stairs. She also had a problem lifting her left leg to get out of the bath and she suffered pain in her left knee after sitting for any length of time. The only way to relieve this was to flex the hip. Alice said she had tired easily for 10 years or so and she felt depressed at times. Her blood pressure was high and pills were controlling it.

X-rays of the hip showed that it was almost normal. However, on examination, there was bad spasm in both her thoracic and lumbar spine. Alice had eight treatments on her back and hip at the end of which time her general health was much better. She stopped feeling depressed and her hip was no longer painful except occasionally after going down stairs. Her blood pressure required about half the number of pills.

Unfortunately, if the joint has become badly worn in the meantime, when the recovery rate is exceeded by wear, treatment to conserve the joint is no longer effective. The amount of wear is usually best assessed on an X-ray and the amount of roughness felt in the joint when moving it by hand.

### Why the diagnosis can be missed
Early arthritis in the hip joint can be very painful but, as with Alice, the diagnosis is often missed. There are three good reasons for this:

■ **Normal X-rays.** For some years, X-rays of the hip joint may not show anything abnormal. The original trouble is probably inflammation of the lining of the joint and the soft tissues, which is followed later by wear of the cartilage of the joint surfaces. Normally, wear is repaired as it takes place. If there is back trouble present, this wear is not fully restored each time, so there is a cumulative effect.

After, say, a year or so, some factor – such as sudden extra exercise or a jolt to the joint – alerts the ganglion to the fact that it has allowed repair to fall very far behind so it presses the alarm button for an emergency repair. This inflammatory reaction is associated with pain, which can be severe. The inflammation often spreads beyond the original area and, in the case of the hip, can affect the two big nerves that pass close to the joint, the sciatic and femoral nerves.

None of this shows up on X-rays, although excessive wear of the cartilage can be deduced by the lessening of the joint space. Deformity and increase in the bone tend not to come on until much later. Of course, the time scale varies a great deal from one person to another.

■ **Misleading distribution of pain.** A disproportionate amount of pain is often felt in the buttocks, down the leg, and even in the knee. Inflammation of the sciatic (see figure 8.5) and femoral nerves causes impulses to be sent to the brain and although these originate at the hip joint, the brain identifies the pain as coming from the sensors at the end of the nerve in these other sites.

The large sciatic nerve is the usual one to become inflamed. It runs across the back of the hip joint right down the leg to the toes. Referred pain from the hip tends to go down to the knees only but,

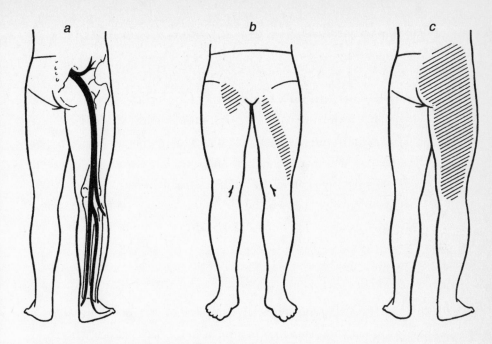

*Figure 8.5* Inflammation of the large sciatic nerve is a common cause of hip pain. Diagram *a* indicates the sciatic nerve; diagram *b* shows the distribution of pain when hip arthritis is mild. Pain may also occur in the buttock; diagram *c* illustrates where hip pain can be experienced when the trouble is severe.

if very severe, it can spread as far as the foot. However, hip arthritis is a less common cause of sciatica than a nerve root being squeezed by a facet joint.

The femoral nerve runs in front of the joint and goes down as far as the knee. This nerve becomes involved less frequently, but when it does, the pain may be in the groin only or radiate from the groin down to the inside of the knee. Intermittent pain in the groin area alone may be present for some years and it will be especially bad after exercising the hip joint. Patients presenting with a pain in the knee should always have the hip investigated.

Pain in the buttock is sometimes due to a cramp in one of the

gluteal (bottom) muscles and so the pain is not associated with the
hip joint.

■ **Pain in the lumbar region.** As we have seen, disabilities in the
upper half of the back may be symptomless for some time but a
problem in the lumbar spine makes itself felt earlier because this area
of the back carries more weight and does more work. Thus, when
someone has had pain in the lumbar region for some years and then
begins to have pain down the leg, the diagnosis of a prolapsed disc
is tempting, although, in fact, the origin may well be in the hip.

---

ATTACK ON TWO FRONTS

To make the situation even more complicated, it is not unusual to
have two sources of referred pain, one from the back because a nerve
root is squeezed in the neural canal, and the other from the
inflamed hip. The inflammation of the nerve root in the back makes
the rest of the nerve very much more sensitive – a light squeeze on
the calf muscle can seem agonizingly painful. It follows then that
what may have been a hardly noticeable problem in the hip joint
can be greatly magnified, causing the pain there to be unbearable.

---

When you know best

Curiously, people with arthritis of the hip often suggest that their
problem may arise from the hip joint but their doctors may insist that
it is a slipped disc. It is usually easy to distinguish between the two:

■ **When the pain lies in the hip joint,** you will often remember
feeling an ache in the groin at infrequent intervals for maybe a year

or so before the real trouble starts. Pain is felt in the buttock and down the leg to the knee. In severe cases, pain can radiate down as far as the foot. It is also common to feel it in the front of the thigh radiating some way down from the groin towards the inner side of the knee.

Hip pain is often improved by walking but may return after a certain distance as the walking starts to irritate the joint. Sitting often produces pain. This is because the joint and the sciatic nerve, which is stretched across the back of the joint, take the weight and the pressure irritates the nerve. The pain may also limit the range of hip movements. It may especially affect the action of putting the leg out sideways and rotating the foot. Hip pain tends to come on gradually over many months.

■ **Pain referred from the back** is often predominantly in the lower part of the leg, especially in the foot and calf (see figure 8.6). There may be numbness in the area. Hip movements are usually normal but you may find it difficult to lift the leg with a straight knee. When lying on your back, the leg should lift almost to a right angle. If the back is pinching the nerve root, there will be agonizing pain down the back of the leg when it is lifted from 10 degrees upwards. Standing, sitting and especially driving tend to aggravate the leg pain. Pain from the back usually comes on very rapidly, within hours or days.

Both types of pain are usually bad during the night and are often improved by exercise. The reason, of course, is that the poor muscle pump during the night allows pressure in the area to increase. This interferes with the tissue circulation and starves the muscles of oxygen, leading to cramps. As soon as you get up and move around, the pressure is reduced and the pain improves.

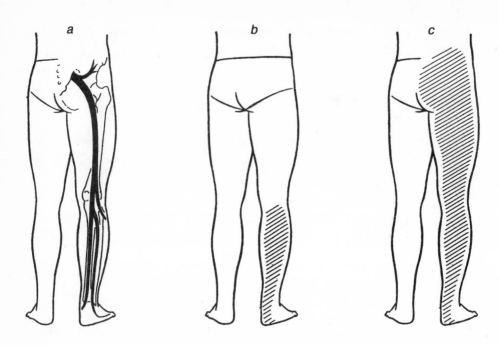

*Figure 8.6* Various kinds of pain in the leg may have their basis in the back when pressure is applied to a nerve root. Diagram *a* shows the sciatic nerve, which is made up of many roots in the lower back; diagram *b* illustrates where referred pain is often felt when there is nerve root involvement; diagram *c* shows how the pain may be distributed in severe cases.

### How back treatment helps

Treatment to the back results in the muscle in spasm returning to normal so the muscle pump is restored. The lumbar ganglion therefore, being dried out, begins to work better at organizing the repair of the hip. Treatment to the joint itself, which is designed to improve the tissue circulation and lessen the spasm of the muscles across the joint, will speed up the effect of the treatment, as will anti-inflammatory pills.

## ARTHRITIS OF THE KNEE

The usual story of arthritis of the knee contrasts markedly with that of the hip. If you twist your knee, it may become painful and sometimes swollen. It clears up only for the trouble to recur with attacks of pain that become more and more frequent.

Treatment to the knee may be enough to redress the balance in a number of cases but for the majority of people, treatment of the back is also needed for permanent relief. This treatment restores the lumbar sympathetic ganglion to working order so it can effectively monitor repair of the joint. Of course, in some cases, the knee's internal cartilage is damaged, but a failure of the repair mechanism due to a malfunction of the ganglion is usually the cause of the problem. Broken off pieces of debilitated cartilage may need surgical removal, but treatment to the back is also needed if the knee is to return to normal.

Another common cause is chronic tonsillitis. Bacteria living in damaged tonsils can put a toxin into the blood that devitalizes any other membranes in the body that are similar to those in the throat. The membrane around a joint is particularly susceptible to this, especially if the joint is already slightly damaged.

---

James, a 17-year-old student, was brought to see me with a swollen and painful left knee that caused him to limp. He thought that he had twisted it during a game of football some months before. It had been uncomfortable after the game and moderately painful the next day. His knee recovered after five days but two months later the pain returned for no obvious reason. The attacks became more frequent and severe until the last one, which had started 10 days before.

His mother said that he had been having sore throats for many years but these had been much less frequent recently. The knee trouble, however, did coincide with the sore throats. On examination, his tonsils were large and unhealthy, although a culture only produced bacteria harmless for the throat. I recommended that the tonsils should be removed. James agreed with my advice, his tonsils were removed, and I gave him some treatment with ultrasonic waves to the lymph nodes in his neck, which were enlarged and inflamed as a result of the long-standing tonsillitis. I was sure that the tonsils were the cause of his painful knee and, as with many other patients, removing them did the trick. His knee slowly improved – with the help of some additional ultrasonic waves and exercise – until it was finally restored to normal after about three months.

It is very common for chronic tonsil infection to cause arthritic joints, a fact that often escapes the attention of diagnosing doctors.

## ARTERIAL DISEASES IN THE LEGS

The lumbar is the lowest of the sympathetic ganglia and it controls the flow of blood through the arteries of the lower part of the body. Its malfunction can have various effects on the legs. For instance, a number of people suffering from lumbar pain complain of a sensation of cold, or sometimes heat, in the leg, but a more serious condition is intermittent claudication. In this case, the artery is diseased and tends to go into a spasm during exercise, making any further movement painful. This is greatly aggravated by the excessive fluid in the region. Once the back has been treated and the underlying problem relieved, there is usually a marked improvement in the distance you can walk without getting severe pain in the calf.

## CAN ANYTHING BE DONE TO HELP?

Although the symptoms I have described in this chapter are usual for these particular disorders, they may vary considerably and it is not practical to go into all the permutations here. However, I hope that enough information has been given for you to be able to distinguish the various diseases from one another.

The preceding chapters have given an account of many of the problems associated with a back that has been injured. Interesting as it may be to study the causes of these problems, the only real concern to sufferers is, 'Can anything be done to help me?'

In the final phase of this book you will find many of the various treatments available to back sufferers together with a detailed description of the method I have devised – although it may not always give permanent relief, it has helped almost every sufferer to return to a normal life.

Before that, however, let's look at the part played by the stellate ganglion in heart disease, and consider how physical treatment to the back can help in the management and prevention of heart problems.

# 9 HEART PROBLEMS AND YOUR BACK

## A new concept in the cause and treatment of coronary thrombosis

To most people, coronary thrombosis seems a straightforward affair – an artery supplying the heart muscle becomes blocked by a clot, the heart suffers shock and may go into major dysfunction and, in the end, the heart and the victim will recover or not, according to the circumstances. But on closer inspection, it is not as simple as that.

- Why, when the severity of arterial disease remains at a constant level, does someone have a heart attack at three o'clock in the morning, then another several months later? How can these periods between attacks be accounted for when the level of disease in the arterial wall remains unchanged?
- Why are other arteries in the body, just as diseased as the coronary artery, hardly ever subject to a thrombosis?
- Why is it that, occasionally, test results for people who have suffered a massive heart attack, even the electro-cardiogram (ECG), can be completely normal? This would not be the case if a permanent clot had been the cause.
- Why, in some instances, does a myocardial infarct – the death of part of the heart muscle because the blood supply to it has been cut off (commonly called a heart attack) – *precede* a coronary thrombosis? Sometimes, in the post-mortem, the clot in the coronary artery is found to have formed after the death of the patient and

thus could not have caused the fatal attack.

■ Why do patients show signs such as tiredness, transient dizziness and indigestion for several years before a coronary thrombosis – and yet all tests are normal?

A simple clot in a coronary artery does not explain any of these phenomena. A spasm of the artery can explain some of them, but not, for instance, why the patient feels ill long before the attack. Tracing the cause of the artery going into a spasm leads, via the nerves transmitting impulses, to one of the controlling nerve centres, our old friend the stellate ganglion. This can provide the answers to these anomalies (see 'Your coronary questions answered', pages 198–206).

## THE MIRACLE PUMP

The heart is an amazingly sophisticated piece of equipment for supplying the body with energy. Indeed, its mechanics are so clever that they are easy to take for granted. Some years ago, a junior minister of power mentioned to me that he was studying alternative methods of obtaining energy for when oil and coal ran out. He described several very elaborate and costly methods of using the Earth's resources, including drilling a hole three miles deep in Cornwall, pouring water on to the red-hot rocks at the bottom and getting back enough steam for a generator to produce sufficient electricity to light a few houses.

Rather tongue in cheek, I replied that this didn't seem a very economical way of solving the problems of the future. Wouldn't it be a more profitable line of research to look into a pump that I knew about? This pump works on a dilute sugar solution for its energy and is capable of filling an average-sized bath in about four minutes.

What's more, the pump itself and enough fuel for about three weeks could be contained in a tin considerably smaller than a one-gallon petrol can. The minister was rather taken aback and said that he was sure no such pump existed because, if it did, he would know all about it. Then I told him which pump I was talking about – the heart.

## CORONARY ARTERIES

The heart is almost entirely made up of muscle known as the myocardium (from the Greek 'myos' meaning muscle, and 'kardia' meaning heart). Like every muscle in the body, it needs a rich supply of blood, especially as, unlike most other muscles, it has to work continuously throughout a person's life. It cannot utilize the blood being pumped through the heart – this blood is too far away from the muscle fibres to service them. In any case, half the blood is being pumped *to* the lungs, having just returned from supplying the body, and therefore contains little oxygen.

So the heart gets its supply of blood through the coronary arteries. The name is very descriptive. Coronary comes from the Latin word 'corona', meaning crown, and these arteries encircle the heart just like a crown. Two arteries branch from the big main artery, the aorta, almost immediately after the latter emerges from the heart, and then divide into a network of smaller branches covering the surface of the heart and running deep into it to supply every muscle fibre with oxygen and essential nutrients. The heart is relatively small in size – little larger than a clenched fist – compared to the work it does. Thus, the coronary arteries are correspondingly shorter in length than those that supply longer and larger muscles (see figure 9.1).

Despite their smaller size, the coronary arteries have to work far

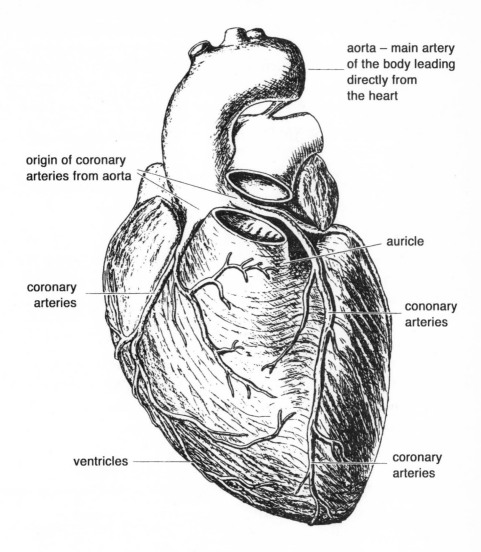

aorta – main artery
of the body leading
directly from
the heart

origin of coronary
arteries from aorta

auricle

coronary
arteries

cononary
arteries

ventricles

coronary
arteries

*Figure 9.1* The heart, showing the coronary arteries.

harder than other arteries in the body because the heart requires such
tremendously differing quantities of blood. To keep pace with these
changes, the coronary arteries are capable of extremely fine-tuning in

controlling the size of their inner diameter – dilating (widening) to increase the supply of blood to the heart and narrowing to decrease it (see figure 9.2). This precise control of the flow of blood through the coronary arteries is monitored by local reactions and, overall, by the stellate ganglion at the base of the neck, the uppermost nerve centre of the sympathetic nerve system.

## WHEN THINGS GO WRONG

When your heart is working well, you probably give it very little thought because it does its job so efficiently. You could compare the heart and its control mechanisms to the smooth-running engine of a luxury car and your body to the framework. It's a rather sad fact of life that, in most cases, you only start to appreciate this beautiful piece of machinery when things go wrong.

A car is a complex mechanism that has many interrelated parts, each dependent on the other to function properly. Any of these parts can go wrong. The fault could be in the engine itself or it may be caused by outside factors such as putting the wrong fuel in the tank, reckless driving or too heavy a load exerting too much of a strain. It may be an amalgamation of different factors. So it is with the heart and its control mechanisms.

It is beyond the scope of this book to examine all the possible causes of heart problems, but it is useful to look at the main things that can go wrong. Broadly speaking, heart trouble can be subdivided into chronic (lasting over a period of time) and acute disease (producing sudden and severe symptoms).

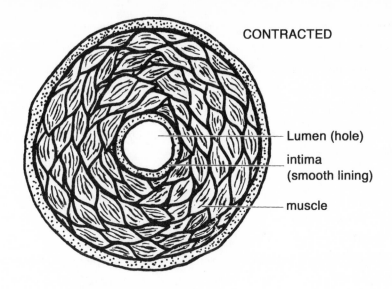

CONTRACTED

Lumen (hole)

intima
(smooth lining)

muscle

*Figure 9.2a* Constricted (narrowed) artery.

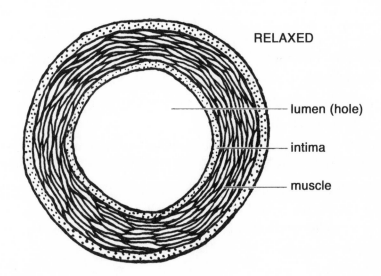

RELAXED

lumen (hole)

intima

muscle

*Figure 9.2b* Dilated (widened) coronary artery.

Chronic heart disease

This is when your heart doesn't work as well as it should. There may be no symptoms for many years as the heart is able to compensate to an amazing extent for a defect. To cope with the extra workload its muscles often overdevelop, thus enlarging the whole heart. When the heart is no longer able to manage any more, one of two things may happen.

- **Congestive heart failure.** The heart is no longer able to pump blood back as fast as it is being used, so fluid begins to collect in the body, causing swelling of the ankles and other parts.
- **Rapid heart failure.** Suddenly unable to cope, the series of events associated with congestive heart failure take place within days.

---

PURPLE FOXGLOVES

It is said that, in the 1780s, a doctor in Shropshire, who was suffering from congestive heart failure, was told that local healers gave patients foxglove leaves to chew to combat the symptoms of the disease. Being in no state to argue, the doctor tried them himself and gave an infusion made from them to his own heart patients. He was amazed how well it worked. This is how the medicinal properties of the purple foxglove (*Digitalis purpurea*) are supposed to have been discovered. The active ingredient found in the foxglove has remained the linchpin of treatment for congestive heart failure to the present day.

MAIN CAUSES OF CHRONIC HEART DISEASE

■ **Valve disorders.** The efficient pumping of the heart depends on four sets of non-return valves, which ensure that blood flows in one direction only. Two valves allow blood into the two sides of the heart but prevent it returning into the veins when the heart pumps; the other two allow blood out of the heart into the arteries but prevent it from regurgitating as the heart fills. Congenital deformation of the valve cusps – the flaps that open to let blood through – results in a faulty valve, as does rheumatic fever, which distorts the valves. If a valve is not working properly, depending on the severity of the situation, blood will leak back to some degree. A defective valve may also interfere with the normal pumping mechanism.

■ **Diminishing elasticity of the arterial walls.** An artery is rather like an elastic balloon, expanding to absorb the surge of blood pumped by the heart throughout its branches and then gradually contracting until the next beat. This converts the pulsing of the heart output into a smooth steady supply of blood to the tissues. If the arteries lose their elasticity due to arterial disease, the fluid pushed through by heartbeat can be accommodated only if there is a significant rise in the pressure from each beat. This means that blood pressure rises. The state of continued high blood pressure is known as hypertension. As the heart makes more and more effort to pump out blood, it will, like all muscles in the body, increase in size to cope with the greater workload. However, there will come a point when it can develop no further and thus will begin to fail.

Acute heart disease

A heart attack is the general name for any sudden cessation of the normal function of the heart. The heart often doesn't stop beating when it has an attack, but it does stop pumping effectively.

Under normal conditions, the muscles in the heart contract from the bottom up, to diminish the size of the ventricles in a co-ordinated action thus achieving the maximum squeezing effect (see figure 9.3). This is brought about by a flat band of specially adapted muscle that radiates from the heart's own pacemaker to all the heart muscle. It regulates the muscle contractions so that their progressive effort make the most effective expulsion of the blood into the blood vessels.

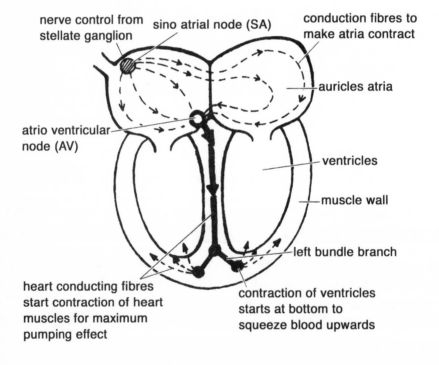

*Figure 9.3* The heart. Transmitting fibres and bundles.

Immediately after it has contracted, the muscle fibres go into a resting phase during which they cannot be stimulated, and it is then that the heart refills before the next contraction takes place.

Straight after a heart attack, the muscle contractions often go round and round the heart without any pattern at all. By the time one wave has passed right round, the muscles have come out of the resting phase and can be stimulated again, so the contraction starts another futile round. Thus, the heart makes hundreds of mini-contractions, none of which do anything in the way of pumping. This is called *ventricular fibrillation*. As a result, blood does not get forced out of the heart to supply the heart muscles, the body or the brain.

## IMPORTANCE OF RESUSCITATION

The brain is a very delicate instrument, and if it is deprived of blood for more than about four minutes, it is likely to suffer irreversible damage. Muscle is less vulnerable to an oxygen shortage, so the heart will survive much longer, continuing its futile contractions. It is vital that a heart-attack victim's blood be kept circulating. Cardio-pulmonary resuscitation (CPR) – the kiss of life plus heart massage – if performed for long enough, ensures that oxygen continues to reach the brain, preventing damage to it. The heart will often resume, or be made to resume, its proper function and the contractions will become adequate again. The defibrillator works by giving a shock to all the muscle fibres at once, putting them into the resting phase. This halts all contractions so that when the pacemaker resumes the heart may well revert to its normal beat. It may, in a number of patients, revert on its own accord, which is why it is so important, in the absence of a defibrillator, to try and maintain a circulation to the brain to give the heart a chance. It has been estimated that some 20,000 people die every year who could have been saved if someone present had known what to do at the time of the attack (see Appendix IV, page 270).

If the heart muscle is deprived of blood for a short time only, the person may make a complete recovery. More commonly, he or she will survive but with partial damage to the heart muscle. The temporary lack of oxygen will kill some of the muscle – hence the term myocardial infarct, which means 'death of heart muscle'. Although this damaged muscle will never recover, it is quite possible to live a perfectly healthy life without it as long as the remainder of the heart is fit and strong. In its prime, the heart muscle has enough power to allow you to run 100 metres in 10 seconds or so. Even when you are older and the heart muscle is not quite so fit, it still has considerable reserves of power. There is plenty left for an average person to lead a normal life.

## WHAT TRIGGERS A HEART ATTACK?

- **Blockage of the blood supply to the heart.** This is the most common cause of heart attacks in middle to later life. If the heart is suddenly deprived of its supply of blood, it will go into complete disarray. As we have seen, the coronary arteries are capable of extremely delicate control of their internal diameters, dilating or narrowing them rapidly to increase or decrease the blood supply as necessary. However, this valuable property makes them vulnerable. If they malfunction, even to a small degree, the supply of blood to the heart can be severely diminished. If the artery is already narrowed through arterial disease, the supply may be closed off completely.

■ **Sudden disruption of the transmitting mechanism in the heart.** This mechanism is responsible for the control and speed of the heartbeat.

■ **Failure of the muscles through toxic interference.** Toxic substances or infections can poison the heart muscle. The heart will continue working as long as possible but when a critical point is reached, heart failure is often almost instantaneous. Among the substances that can have this effect are direct infections of the heart muscle, such as a flu virus, toxins from certain kinds of bacteria that can cause sore throats and, of course, certain poisons.

Infections can invade your body as a whole, attacking all your muscles including your heart. There is a real danger of inducing a fatal muscle failure if you take fairly vigorous exercise too soon after a viral infection, especially flu. If your heart is still in an inflamed and sensitive state, it may not be strong enough to cope with the increase in workload, and it may suddenly go into uncontrolled contractions that could be fatal.

Elizabeth, 23 and extremely fit, died following a flu virus. She was on a skiing holiday with friends in Switzerland when she had an attack of flu. She stayed in bed for three days and took it easy for the next day. By the fifth day, she was so fed up with losing good skiing time that she went out with her friends on an advanced slope. On the way down, she suddenly fell and, when she eventually came to rest, remained motionless. When one of her friends reached her, she was already dead. A post-mortem found that her heart muscles and membranes were inflamed. This was attributed to the virus.

What else can cause problems?

There are many other factors that can interrupt the smooth running of the heart, especially an interruption of the oxygen supply to the lungs or a poison that prevents the blood from carrying it around. Severe loss of blood is another factor. The main risk factors can be divided into those that can be controlled, including an unhealthy diet, lack of exercise, being overweight and smoking, and those that cannot be changed, such as age, heredity, sex (men are more susceptible to heart attacks than women), race and culture. The traditional diets of some peoples, notably the Japanese and Inuit, contain less fat and sugar than western diets and coronary disease is not prevalent among them.

## WHAT CAUSES THE BLOCKAGE?

The most popular idea about what causes a blockage in the heart muscle's blood supply is that a clot forms in the artery completely blocking it, and that this clot comes about because of damage to the wall of the artery from pre-existing disease. More recently, a spasm of the coronary artery has been recognized as a factor in at least some of the cases. So the four main events that can cause a blockage of the blood supply are, in sequence:

– artery narrowed by its nerve control
– artery narrowed by disease in its wall
– arterial spasm further narrowing or closing the artery
– artery blocked by a clot

While accepting that the level of heart disease has a major bearing on the outcome, I believe that what initiates the actual attack is a malfunction of the stellate ganglion, and without this the attack might never have taken place.

## ARTERY NARROWED BY NERVE CONTROL

In a healthy body, the sympathetic nerve chain balances and opposes the parasympathetic. As we have seen in chapter 6, this is rather like a tug-of-war, with each nerve system balancing the other to maintain a state of harmony. If one side increases or decreases its output, the equilibrium is disturbed. If, under normal conditions, the sympathetic nerve system slows down, the parasympathetic responds by becoming more active. If one is stimulated, the other almost switches off. When, for example, the sympathetic is activated through fear, the para-sympathetic almost completely cuts off its output so that energy is not wasted during the crisis.

If the sympathetic drive is low, the internal diameter of the arteries is maintained at a smaller size than normal and, as a result, the heart does not get quite the right amount of oxygen. As the output of the sympathetic nervous system diminishes further, the internal diameter of the arteries becomes increasingly smaller. In the early stages, this may have no noticeable effect but, at a later date, it can give rise to what is known as angina-of-effort, which is felt as a sharp pain in the chest.

---

## FORMS OF ANGINA

As a matter of interest, angina simply means pain. You can have angina in parts of the body other than the heart. If you are suffering from one form of sore throat, for example, this is known as Vincent's angina. If the pain is felt in the chest, it is called angina pectoris (pectoris meaning chest).

---

### Shortage of oxygen

Angina pectoris normally arises when a person takes some form of exercise or is particularly excited or anxious about something. The heart works harder and the muscles require an increased supply of blood. If the blood flow through the coronary arteries is diminished, the heart cannot get enough blood to supply its muscles with the required amount of oxygen. Like all muscles, the heart muscles become painful when short of oxygen, so the person experiences a fearful pain in the chest – and the left arm.

The pain is very sharp indeed, like a cramp in your leg although in that case the pain is actually felt in the calf muscle. In the case of the heart, things are slightly different. The heart shares a sensory nerve supply with the wall of the chest and down the left arm. Our hearts are almost always very strong and work for many years without any problems, so if anything goes wrong, the brain assumes that it is the chest and/or the arm that are malfunctioning, not the reliable old war-horse in your chest. For this reason, the pain is felt as a vice-like sensation around the chest and down the arm, and not in the heart itself.

The pain experienced by a person during an angina attack usually goes after a few minutes' rest as the muscles recover, but it comes back again after another bout of exercise.

Keith, a 53-year-old barber, came to me complaining that he could walk about 100 metres (330ft) before he got a severe pain in the chest, which he described as 'clamp-like', and found it difficult to breathe. After a rest, he was able to resume his walk until he had the pain again. He had been investigated and just a slight narrowing of his coronary arteries had been found. He was advised to continue with an artery-dilating drug, which gave him complete relief at the time.

However, the painful attacks had started up again and were becoming more frequent. Keith said he was getting worried and wanted my opinion. He said he tired easily and had a lot of fibrositis between his shoulders following a whiplash injury nine years previously. In addition, he had been treated for a gastric ulcer some years before.

On examination I was able to trace the root of the problem. It lay in his spinal column and was causing an upset in the sympathetic balance in his system, giving rise to the angina and other health problems. After a total of 14 sessions over a period of 14 months, he has remained symptom-free for several years. Keith also says that he has more energy, less digestive trouble and feels far better in himself.

For Keith, angina pectoris was an early warning that something was amiss in his body. The situation can get progressively worse until it reaches a point where coronary arteries are too narrow to allow a sufficient blood supply to nourish the muscles under everyday working conditions.

## ARTERY NARROWED BY DISEASE IN ITS WALL

All the arteries in the body, including the coronary arteries, can be affected by *atherosclerosis* – a plaque, which is a deposit of fibrous material, forming in the artery walls. The plaque can damage and even kill an artery's muscle and elastic tissue by pressing on it, replacing it with more fibrous tissue. These degenerative changes occur within the arterial wall, and fatty deposits start to appear under the inner lining. Any artery in the body can be affected and symptoms seldom arise. It is virtually only in the coronary and cerebral (brain) arteries that crises can occur.

In the coronary arteries, atherosclerosis causes heart attacks; in the cerebral arteries, it causes strokes. More than half of a normal artery can be closed through atherosclerosis, which means almost all of it can be blocked when the artery contracts. This narrowing may not matter so much in a small artery that does not supply a large volume of heart muscle. However, in a large artery, it is likely to cause a major heart attack.

## ARTERIAL SPASM FURTHER NARROWING OR CLOSING THE ARTERY

We have already seen that a low sympathetic drive will result in a modest, continuing narrowing of the artery wall. During exercise, this may cause the pain of angina because the muscle is not getting sufficient oxygen. A sudden drop in the sympathetic drive can cause the artery to go into a spasm, closing it partially or completely. This will cut off the blood supply to the heart muscle, causing an attack similar to a thrombosis.

One of three things will result:

- The artery may reopen reasonably rapidly before any damage to the heart muscle takes place and the person will maybe suffer a momentary dizzy spell and then recover completely.
- The artery remains in spasm and the person could die with no clot present.
- When the artery is in spasm, a clot forms at the site of arterial disease and this will block off the artery semi-permanently,

resulting in a heart attack with some death of the muscle supplied by the artery.

The effects of the spasm are obviously much more serious in a diseased artery because it is already narrowed and the special smooth lining that prevents clotting will be roughened. This combined with the reduced blood flow will readily result in a clot forming, leading to a heart attack. If the victim survives, the heart muscle that has actually died will gradually form fibrous tissue to keep the heart wall intact. This patch can sometimes slowly start to bulge under the pressure of the blood in the ventricle at each contraction, and occasionally such scar tissue actually bursts, causing death.

## ARTERY BLOCKED BY A CLOT

Clots can get into the coronary system and lodge in an artery, thus blocking it. However, this is rare. There are few sources of such clots. All the blood from the body goes through the lungs, which act as a very fine filter, and therefore the clot has to come from somewhere beyond the lungs. There are two possibilities – it either breaks off from a diseased valve, or it breaks off from a clot on the wall of a damaged larger coronary artery and blocks a smaller branch further down.

## MALFUNCTION OF THE STELLATE GANGLION

On its own, arterial disease is seldom the cause of heart attacks. A poorly operating stellate ganglion is the crux of the problem.

Among other functions, this nerve centre controls the amount of blood passing through the arteries to the brain and to the heart. A malfunction may upset the supply of blood to the heart – but if it does, it does not do so when it has a problem. Indeed, it will be subject to malfunction for a long time before the coronary arteries are affected if they are at all. This may be due to two reasons:

– The stellate ganglion controls various parts of the body and so something going wrong may give rise to a number of different ailments. A disruption may, for example, cause a spasm of the arteries to the brain, causing a migraine, or it may affect the arteries to the hands, leading to Raynaud's disease, or it could affect the supply of blood through the coronary arteries to the heart. The reason why one of these is predominant may be partly genetic – an hereditary sensitivity of the ganglion in its control of various parts of the body – or it may be due to the fact that the weakest link is the part most easily affected.

– The heart is one of the body's most primitive parts, extremely tough and hard to upset. The more primitive an organ is, the less likely it is to be affected if the sophisticated controls in the body go wrong. There has to be a major disturbance of the sympathetic drive before the heart can be affected. Even when you are deeply unconscious, the control over your breathing and the pumping of your heart continues.

The heart is one of the last organs controlled by the stellate ganglion to be affected by any disruption. It is important that this point is fully understood to prevent false alarms – a twinge in the base of the neck does not mean that you are about to have a heart attack!

Reaching crisis point

As the congestion around the stellate ganglion increases, the situation will become worse. The cumulative effects of the poor circulation in the area eventually reach such a critical point that the stellate ganglion suddenly withdraws its support almost completely. As the sympathetic pull on a coronary artery lessens, so the parasympathetic system reacts by contracting the muscles of the artery wall and eventually causing it to go into spasm, resulting in a partial or complete blockage of the blood supply to the heart muscle.

This critical point takes several hours, even days, to reach from the first major drop in the sympathetic drive. However, those affected will almost certainly have been suffering to some extent from the symptoms of a low sympathetic drive for a number of years.

---

Alice, aged 57, was a moderately well-known actress. She had been feeling off-colour for two days and on the third felt bad enough to see her doctor. She had seen him already some months previously because her indigestion had become worse, but this had rapidly cleared with medication. The doctor now decided that she was run down and advised her to take at least a day off. Unfortunately, the demanding producer she was working for was not satisfied that she was actually ill, so it was decided that 'the show must go on'.

In the middle of the second act, she suddenly felt dizzy and fainted; her understudy took her place. She had had a minor coronary thrombosis, and she was off work for several months.

---

This is a very common story. People very often feel tired or unwell for anything from one to three days before a coronary attack. The crisis can be brought about by a number of factors:

- **Anxiety and worry** over such things as business difficulties can make you tighten all your muscles as if ready for a fight, especially those in the neck and shoulder area, thus diminishing the muscle pump and increasing congestion. This is what happened to Alice when she went on stage.

- **Complete rest** also diminishes the workings of the muscle pump. If the activity of the pumping mechanism is already poor due to muscle spasm, a period of rest could reduce it almost to a standstill. Then the congestion in the area becomes too great for the stellate ganglion to cope with. It is for this reason that many people suffer coronary attacks in the early hours of the morning after several hours of complete rest.

- **Unaccustomed exercise** can generate heart problems. By the time people reach their 40s, they may be taking little exercise, and the muscles around the stellate ganglion have fewer demands for oxygen. Circulation is maintained at a low, but adequate level. As soon as that person gets involved in vigorous exercise, such as a game of squash or a hard run, the muscles need more oxygen, so the blood circulating locally rapidly increases. If there is spasm of the muscles present, the congestion gets worse until there will come a point when, due to lack of oxygen and the build-up of waste products, the stellate ganglion will malfunction, causing a sudden coronary spasm.

- **Weather** can have an adverse affect if you are nearing a coronary attack. The particles in the air – dust, pollens, bacteria, moulds and so on – are ionized. Negatively charged ions cause no reaction but positive ions react with the platelets in the blood, causing the liberation of serotonin, one of the brain's chemical transmitters (see page 56).

    Serotonin has a profound effect on almost all of the body – it causes it to become congested, with the result that more fluid than normal diffuses into the tissues. Any area already congested becomes even more so. Symptoms may appear if there were none before and existing ones may be made worse.

■ **Smoking** paralyses some nerve centres and this makes arteries contract. One puff of smoke and an artery can remain contracted for some minutes.

Severity of the spasm

The spasm may cause a partial blockage of the coronary artery or a complete close-down, followed by a clot that would make the blockage semi-permanent and may be fatal. This is influenced by several factors:

■ **The degree and activity of the disease in the artery**. If the artery is already narrowed by disease, a contraction that was intended, for example, to close the artery down to three-quarters of its diameter may cause a total shutdown. Furthermore, if the disease is recent and active, platelets will stick more readily to the artery walls and there is a higher risk of a clot forming.

■ **The amount that the spasm narrows the artery.** If there is only a minor contraction, there may not be enough stagnant blood to form a clot. The degree of spasm directly corresponds to the degree of malfunction of the stellate ganglion. This, in turn, is influenced by the amount of waterlogging in the area of the neck and thoracic spine, which is affected by the severity of the injury to the back and by external conditions such as the weather.

■ **The duration of the spasm.** If the artery can relax quickly enough, it may well dilate before any, or only a small, clot is formed, especially if there is no disease present in the arterial wall. If the spasm lasts longer, a major clot may form, and this will be followed by a full-blown coronary thrombosis.

## CORONARY QUESTIONS ANSWERED

Several anomalies surrounding heart disease are not easily explained by mainstream theory. To find the answers, we must look beyond the popular theory of arterial disease as the cause of coronary attacks.

*Why do people often feel unwell for up to three days before a heart attack?*

If a sudden clot in the artery is the cause of the attack, how can this preliminary period of illness be accounted for? During the 12 to 24 hours preceding a heart attack, many people go to their doctors complaining of feeling very unwell and that they are unusually tired and tensed up. They are generally advised to stop work and take things easy.

Anthony, who was 63 and very active, had suffered from aches between his shoulders on and off for about 12 years. One Tuesday morning he was feeling so off-colour and tired that he went to see his GP, who examined him but found nothing abnormal. The doctor told Anthony to take it easy for a day or so.

That evening, Anthony felt so much better he went to see some friends. As the evening went on, he started to have bad attacks of indigestion and then a pain in his left shoulder and arm. He suddenly collapsed unconscious and his friends called an ambulance. When he arrived at hospital, it was found that he had suffered a coronary attack and he was taken to intensive care. Thankfully, he survived.

It is my belief that when someone like Anthony feels unwell, the possibility that this might be a precursor to a heart attack should always be considered. The person may be suffering from a sudden sharp drop in the sympathetic drive, which is about to reach the critical point giving rise to a spasm of a coronary artery.

*Why is it that when someone who has just suffered a massive heart attack arrives at hospital, the tests – even an ECG – can be completely normal?*

If a clot has caused the coronary blockage, it will still be present, shutting off the blood supply to a part of the heart muscle. The damage to the heart will be considerable. The ECG will detect the effect of the clot on the pumping action of the muscle, and blood tests will detect any products of the breaking up of muscles. When a muscle is damaged, some of it dies and proteins are released as it disintegrates. The level of these breakdown products can be measured to assess the degree of damage to the heart muscle.

---

Peter, a 49-year-old solicitor, was sitting at his desk when he suffered a bad attack of pain on the left side of his chest and down his left arm. He went straight to hospital, but his ECG and blood tests were all normal. However, the pain had been so severe that he was put on a coronary regime.

The trouble soon subsided, but five months later, he felt the pains again and he went to hospital. The results were the same – no signs of abnormality in his ECG or his blood tests.

On his third attack, he came to me and I found that he had tremendous spasm of the upper thoracic paravertebral muscles and a very tender second thoracic vertebra. After six sessions of treatment, Peter said he had not felt so well in a very long time. Six years later, the pains have still not recurred.

Why did all of Peter's tests show normal results? The answer is that the blockage was caused by a spasm of the coronary artery that had subsided by the time he reached hospital. In such a case as Peter's, there was too little disease in the artery to make it vulnerable to a thrombosis, so the muscle remained completely undamaged.

*Most arteries in the body are prone to disease, so why is it usually only the coronary and cerebral arteries that cause any trouble?*

If disease alone causes blockages in arteries, many of our arteries would be as vulnerable to a thrombosis as the coronary and cerebral arteries. Other factors must be involved.

The coronary and cerebral arteries differ from other arteries in that their role requires them to change their internal diameters rapidly and with amazing precision from being very dilated to being very small. If other arteries are diseased, there is usually still plenty of room for blood to pass through, even in their most contracted state. However, with a coronary artery, it takes only a small amount of disease and then a spasm to close it off completely, thus running the risk of a clot.

Sarah, a 57-year-old designer, considered herself to be of average fitness, although she took little exercise. One morning at breakfast, she suddenly felt ill with a severe pain in her chest and numbness in her left shoulder, which radiated a little into her left arm. She was taken to hospital but died the next day.

The post-mortem examination showed a thrombosis in one of her coronary arteries. There was atherosclerosis at the site of the thrombosis, but this was slight and almost certainly not enough in itself to have caused the clot.

*It is known that arterial disease comes on slowly and remains relatively constant. Yet people often recover from one attack and lead perfectly normal lives only to suffer another attack several months later. If there is enough disease to cause a thrombosis on one day, how do you account for the periods between attacks when the level of disease remains unchanged?*

The answer is that a blockage of the artery is not caused solely by disease but is the result of a spasm of a diseased artery. The story of one of my patients who subsequently became a great friend illustrates this anomaly.

Mike, a 58-year-old stockbroker, had 14 heart attacks in the space of three years. Soon after his third attack, he was advised to retire as it was likely that he would suffer another one in the near future. Mike ignored this advice. He came to me after his 14th attack, saying he was at his wits' end. He didn't want to give up work but he was seriously worried about his health – why did the attacks keep recurring?

During his first visit, I felt a spasm from the back of his skull to the vertebrae in his lower back. He said that he became tired very easily and always seemed to feel tensed up. He had fibrositis between his shoulders and had suffered from indigestion for about 15 years.

Mike had such a low sympathetic drive that it was causing spasms of the coronary artery. I gave him treatment over three months, with 14 visits in all, after which he felt so well that he continued with his job, dying of pneumonia 21 years later, aged 79, having had no further heart problems.

*Many heart attacks occur in the early hours of the morning. If the level of disease is constant day and night, how can this be explained?*

To answer that we need to take another look at the muscle pump, which circulates blood back to the heart. This mechanism is activated by movement of the muscles. In a healthy body at rest, adequate circulation is maintained by a combination of the residual pressure from the heart, waves of contractions up the vein walls and the minimal movements that a person makes when asleep. However, if the person already has a spasm of the muscles of the back, causing oedema in the tissues, prolonged rest can cause a sufficient increase in the tissue fluid to result in a crisis of the sympathetic nerve system. This would give rise to a spasm of the coronary artery.

---

Simon, 42, was a large man who had been out of work for several years. He was very tense about financial problems and tried to relax by taking a lot of exercise. He had bouts of indigestion and got tired very easily, symptoms which he put down to his difficult circumstances.

Then one night at about 2.45 a.m., he awoke with a bad attack of indigestion. He tried taking antacids but the pain in his stomach became worse, and after about three-quarters of an hour, he sent for a doctor. His pulse was weak and his blood pressure low. On reaching hospital, an ECG confirmed that he had had a coronary thrombosis. He was in hospital for three weeks.

---

*Why does a post-mortem sometimes show that a myocardial infarct precedes a coronary thrombosis?*

There have been several occasions when pathologists have found that a thrombosis formed after a patient died and was thus not the cause of death.

This happened to Freda, the 51-year-old mother of three teenagers. Much to the great distress of the family, Freda died suddenly at home. When her body was examined at post-mortem, a clot was found in one of the coronary arteries. However, this was deemed to have come about after her death when the stationary blood reacted with some roughening of the artery wall. This obviously meant that the clot could not have caused the fatal attack.

So what was the cause? The answer was that Freda had such a depleted sympathetic drive that it caused the coronary artery to go into spasm. As the artery was already narrowed by disease, this spasm was enough to close off the blood supply to the heart muscle causing death of heart muscle. The formation of the clot occurred as a natural sequence of events after Freda died. The fatal stoppage of blood was caused by the spasm, not the thrombosis.

*Why do some cardiac patients have histories of transient dizzy spells for several years before the heart attacks?*

There are, of course, many common causes of dizziness, but if none of these is diagnosed, the possibility of low sympathetic drive should be considered.

Harry, a 49-year-old postman, had had a mild heart attack. He told me that he had been seeing doctors for about 12 years because he had dizzy spells. These lasted for several minutes, came on at different times of the day and didn't seem to be brought on by anything special. Investigations had not shown any particular cause. However, an ECG revealed signs of previous slight damage to the heart muscle, and the dizzy spells were thought to have been very minor heart attacks.

My view of Harry's medical history is that he had been suffering from low sympathetic drive. This had caused a number of minor spasms of one of his coronary arteries, which had been enough to make his heart falter and cause the dizzy spells, but not enough to give rise to any serious problem. Then his sympathetic drive finally dropped enough, or the spasm lasted long enough, to cause a minor heart attack.

*Why should a relatively fit person suffer a heart attack while playing squash or jogging?*

If you watch a squash player or a jogger in action, you will see that the muscles in the neck have to work very hard to hold the head in a stationary position on top of the moving body. Nevertheless, they may not contract and expand enough to generate the greatly increased blood flow they require. This is especially true if there is a great deal of tension involved – a considerable tightening of the shoulder muscles will result in greater congestion of the neck area and will eventually disrupt the stellate ganglion to such an extent that a coronary spasm results.

David, 47, was an active gardener who played regular games of football and squash. He liked to lead life to the full although he did have indigestion and tired very easily once he got home after a day's work.

He was playing squash one evening at about eight o'clock when he complained of a cramp-like pain in his chest and then suddenly collapsed. He was taken to hospital and a coronary thrombosis was diagnosed. After a spell in intensive care, he made a good recovery.

*Statistics show that the peak age for heart attacks is between 40 and 55. How can you account for this?*

The muscles are still strong at this age, especially in men. In addition, many people have injured their backs in the past without realizing it. This is also an age when people become less involved in exercise yet still consider themselves fairly active. They are likely to place a lot of intermittent and unaccustomed demands on their bodies, doing tasks such as chopping wood or moving heavy furniture.

The congestion in the neck area from an old injury would be considerably increased by such activity. The muscles are still powerful, and the increase in the blood supply to meet their needs when exercising can all too easily flood the area. The combination of unaccustomed exercise and a diseased artery makes such a person vulnerable to a coronary episode.

By the age of 65 or so, all the muscles in the body become weaker. It follows that the protective spasm across the facet joints could be correspondingly weaker, and in my experience, there is often a spontaneous improvement in the back's condition. This leads to an easing of the congestion around the stellate ganglion and reduces the risk of a coronary attack.

*The incidence of coronary attacks used to be far higher in men than in women, but the pendulum is starting to swing back. Why is this so?*

Although men are still at the greater risk of a coronary attack, more and more women are becoming vulnerable. This may be because, until some decades ago, women were far less likely to participate in strenuous activities, so their muscles were correspondingly weaker. As a result, the spasm across the facet joints was less intense and the congestion of the back and associated tissues was less severe than in men. Now that more women are taking part in a wide range of competitive sports and keep-fit exercises, they are suffering more injuries and also developing stronger muscles. In these circumstances, one would expect a closing of the gap between the incidence of coronary attacks in the two sexes. The protection of the arteries in women is another reason why I so strongly advocate the use of hormone replacement therapy when needed.

*A number of factors are known to increase the risk of a coronary attack. Yet despite the variety and number of these factors, two-thirds of all people who have attacks have no known risk factor. Why is this?*

To counter this puzzling fact, here's another interesting statistic. The number of people with a back problem who have trouble with their thoracic spine is only slightly more than the number of people suffering coronary attacks – i.e. about 40 per cent of the population, as opposed to 30 per cent having heart attacks. This statistic, which backs up my theory, should not be ignored. When you are dealing with such large numbers of people vulnerable to a serious illness, it is imperative that all avenues be explored in the prevention of attacks.

## MANAGEMENT OF A CORONARY PROBLEM

The care that needs to be given immediately following a coronary episode is outside the scope of this book, other than to emphasize the importance of calling for skilled medical help and learning the resuscitation techniques that could keep a person alive until either this help arrives or the heart resumes an adequate beat (see Appendix IV, page 270). My treatment is not a substitute for conventional, orthodox medicine. The advice and treatment given by cardiologists is of the very highest standard. Recognizing the risks and preventing a first or further attack are my aims and I hope this book will add an extra dimension to the treatment of coronary attacks. My method is focussed on the bruised facet joints and muscle spasms caused by an old injury, and the consequent disruption to the stellate ganglion.

---

The other day, a postcard arrived on my desk from one of my patients on holiday in Norway. 'Never felt better,' she wrote. Twelve months previously, Julie, a 27-year-old air hostess, had come to me with excessive tiredness, indigestion, headaches, bouts of mild depression and fibrositis between her shoulder blades. She had also had a few mild fainting attacks that had lasted several minutes. Julie had been working long hours and didn't think she could cope much longer. Her doctor had been unable to offer positive help.

After a thorough examination, I diagnosed symptoms of low sympathetic drive. I explained that if the underlying condition was not treated, there was a slight risk of a more serious complication. She agreed to treatment and within several months her condition and quality of life had improved dramatically.

If Julie's condition had not been diagnosed, she may have been at risk of a heart attack. By treating the fundamental cause, I was able greatly to reduce this risk (if it had indeed been present) and also improve her general health beyond measure.

## ON A LESS HAPPY NOTE

There have been three occasions when I have seen patients for a small problem and, after listening to their medical histories and examining them, have decided that they were at some risk of a coronary attack. In each case, for differing reasons, they were unable or unwilling to undergo treatment, and each had a coronary thrombosis within the following 18 months.

One was the 64-year-old wife of a neighbour, whom I examined one evening because she had a very painful back. She regarded me simply as 'the gardener next door' and saw little reason to follow my advice. The second was a shopkeeper whose establishment I visited often. He came to me for a consultation because of intermittent back trouble. Despite my warning, he said he was a busy man and it would have to be a major problem before he would come for treatment.

The third patient was a senior administrator at the Royal Homoeopathic Hospital, who consulted me about his painful toe. I examined him and, among other things, found that he had a great deal of oedema at the base of his neck, muscle spasm in this area and a history of several dizzy spells and one momentary blackout over the past few years. I explained that his toe was a relatively easy problem, but he had other trouble that could cause anxiety in a year or two, so he should have treatment as soon as possible to rectify this as well. He said that he was about to make his annual three-month visit to Barbados, and that as soon as he got back, he would take my advice and have treatment. Unfortunately, he never returned to England. Just over two months later, he had a massive coronary attack and died in Barbados.

Thankfully, I cannot remember any other patients who were nearing a critical phase but who refused treatment.

## Beta-blockers

Among the drugs commonly used in the treatment of coronary trouble, beta-blockers damp down the whole sympathetic-adrenalin mechanism. Beta-receptors are the adrenalin-activity-producing part of the sympathetic nervous system. By blocking them, the activity of the sympathetic nervous system is reduced in proportion to the amount of drug given.

There is, however, an anomaly in the use of beta-blockers – if a low sympathetic drive causes a coronary attack, a drug to lower the sympathetic drive further would hardly seem appropriate as a treatment for the attack as it would diminish the diameter of the coronary arteries. But by lowering the whole activity of the body, including the output of the heart muscle, beta-blockers ensure that the heart has a great deal less work to do than normal. This is the all-important consideration, even though the heart's blood supply might be further reduced, as it would already be due to arterial disease or spasm.

Beta-blockers also lower blood pressure, further assisting the heart by cutting its load.

There are a number of beta-blocker drugs and they all have slightly different effects as they work on different parts of the sympathetic nervous system. In addition, the effects of the same drug can be different in different people.

If the stellate ganglion is the centre of the cause of the coronary thrombosis, this is because it is in an area of oedema where the tissue circulation is very poor. For this reason, any drug given by mouth will have little, if any, effect on it. This means that the rest of the body will benefit from the beta-blocker without a major adverse effect on the size of the coronary arteries themselves – i.e. the drug will not decrease the internal diameters of these arteries. So oedema around the stellate ganglion may explain the anomaly of why a drug that is supposed to reduce the diameters of the coronary arteries can actually be of use in the treatment of heart trouble.

---

PHYSICAL MEDICINE

A rule of thumb is that the risk of any treatment must never exceed the risk of not having the treatment. If you have had a coronary attack, some risk might be permissible in an attempt to avoid another one. Fortunately, however, no risk is involved with physical treatment.

---

AIDS TO RECOVERY

Positive attitude of mind

This has a great influence on the ability of your body to repair itself. Just as people are split into those who rejoice that their glass is half full and those who complain that their glass is half empty, so the attitudes of cardiac patients are divided. Some feel lucky to have survived an attack and resolve to stay fit and live a long time, while others feel that the sword of Damocles is suspended by a thread six inches above their heads and spend their life in constant dread of another attack.

Unfortunately, the latter is all too often a self-perpetuating philosophy, but it doesn't always have to be that way.

Mary had suffered a mild coronary thrombosis and was in a very depressed frame of mind. She was worried about how she would cope at home and how she would look after her husband on his return from a business trip to Australia. As her spirits sank deeper and deeper, she seemed to lose all incentive to get better. Thankfully, her husband cut his trip short and was home within a few days. It was touching to see how pleased they were to see each other. As Mary's face lit up, it was as if someone had flicked on an electric light. With her husband's encouragement, she adopted a more positive outlook on life and recovered rapidly.

Normal lifestyle

After recovering from a heart attack, it is important to live as normal a life as possible – much better for morale. When people come to me for treatment, I often suggest that they let up a little on any rigorous regime prescribed by their consultants. If they have been taken off foods or drinks they enjoy, for example, I advise partaking in great moderation. Many people say they feel much better at the mere thought of being able to enjoy a small brandy at the end of the day.

A normal lifestyle is also physically better for you. If you get out and move about more, you keep the muscle pump active and recovery is speeded up. If you lie around in bed or on the sofa and worry, you are hindering your body's natural repair mechanisms.

Many years ago, a great friend of mine had a severe coronary thrombosis at the age of 62. She was the thin, active type who had enjoyed every aspect of life and been very fit until the heart attack struck her down. Imagine, therefore, her dismay when she was told by the foremost heart specialist of the day that, if she wished to see another year, she would have to live the life of a cabbage. She was advised to move her bed to the ground floor of her house to avoid the exertion of stairs, and not to get up until after lunch. She was allowed to potter about in the garden until tea time, after which it would be wise for her to return to bed. The alternative? If she was any more active than this, her prospects for survival may well be just a few weeks.

Following a short conference with her very supportive husband, she decided to go down with all flags flying. A trip to Switzerland was rapidly arranged so that she could fulfil the wish of a lifetime. As a keen gardener, she had always wanted to see the Alpine plants at their best and this was the ideal time of year.

She tramped over the Alps for six weeks and returned with a crate of plants for her own beautiful garden. The following year, she went again, and by the time her heart finally claimed her – after 17 fit and active years – she was reputed to have one of the finest collections of Alpine plants in Britain.

There is a small twist to the story. On the fourth year, she brought back plants for her cardiologist who was also renowned for his garden. When he looked a little annoyed by the present, she said, 'You know, James, you would much rather have sent me flowers to prove that you were correct than receive them from me, which proves that you were wrong in your original advice.'

Support from family and friends

In my practice, spouses are always invited to join the consultation. This is for two reasons. First, they often remember past injuries and early symptoms far better than the patient – 'You had a bad tumble down the stairs the year after we were married,' or 'You complained of a dreadful ache after planting those bulbs four summers ago.' The patient may not feel such information is relevant, but it is most helpful to me.

Second, if the patient's partner and family understand what I am aiming to achieve with the treatment and how it can help prevent future attacks, I can usually rely on them to keep the patient on the straight and narrow. A wife, for example, will remind her husband to do his daily exercises; a husband will ensure that this wife continues coming for treatment until the problem is cleared up. It is so important that families work together to help restore the patient to good health. Sadly, this was not the case with Miles, who always seemed so cheery.

Miles was in hospital. He had had a minor coronary thrombosis followed by pneumonia and pleurisy, but fortunately was making a good recovery. He was the life and soul of the ward, and if any patient was a bit miserable, Miles could be relied upon to be there with a friendly word. Any nurse who was a bit pushed could be sure that help was at hand. Miles told us all about his wonderful family and home. He said that, when his 'super' son Martin had married, Miles had bought a big house and let Martin and his new wife live in it. Miles occupied a bedsitting room, completely self-contained, on the first floor, and said that he enjoyed helping out with the babysitting and shopping.

None of us had met Martin because, for one reason after another, he had never managed to make the journey to the hospital to visit his father. Never mind, said Miles, it would all be made up in the celebrations when at last he returned home. When Miles was well enough, we got in touch with his son to say that he could pick up his father at the end of the week. 'I don't mind what you do with the old fool,' the son said. 'We're sick of his jokes and stupid stories. Find an old people's home or something for him – we'll never have him back here.'

Miles went quiet at the news and just sat silent in his bed. He never really said anything again. He just did not wake up one morning. He had had a massive coronary thrombosis and slipped away into peaceful oblivion. Had he had something to live for, we were all sure that Miles would have continued to spread his own particular brand of sunshine for many more years.

Upsetting though this story is, it is important to remember that the opposite is equally true. Help, support and love encourage patients' own repair mechanisms so that they recover more quickly and completely than they would otherwise have done.

## LOOK OUT FOR THE SIGNS

There are certain symptoms that become very marked in the few days before the congestion in the area of the stellate ganglion reaches crisis point. A very clear clinical picture builds up that you may recognize if you have already suffered a coronary attack, or someone close to you has. It is characterized by the symptoms listed below, which are all signs of a low sympathetic drive. Anyone displaying *all* of these should be checked over. The symptoms do not necessarily mean that a heart attack is imminent, but it is sensible to be checked as a precautionary measure:

- **Aches** between the shoulders or in the neck.
- **Extreme tiredness** which tends to peak at around three in the afternoon. Sufferers tend to have the energy to cope when under pressure, even an ordinary day's work, but become very tired as soon as they relax.
- **Indigestion, headaches and dizzy spells,** and the tendency to get tensed up very easily.

Whether or not these symptoms are indicative of a vulnerability to a heart attack, they deserve treatment in their own right. The majority of my patients say they didn't realize how bad they were feeling before they had the treatment; they had thought that, apart from discomfort, they were perfectly well. It is rather like looking around a room and wondering if it needs decorating. The tendency is to leave it for a year or so. It is only when you have given the room a new coat of paint that you realize how tatty it was before. If your health deteriorates slowly, you won't be aware that it is going downhill because you can't recall what it was like to be normal. It's not until your health is restored that you appreciate just how ill you had been feeling.

Reggie, aged 53, had had a sudden pain in his chest as he hurried after a bus five years previously. Fortunately, it had passed off quickly as soon as he sat down in the bus. He had forgotten all about it and carried on with his life. Unfortunately, not long afterwards, he had had another attack of pain as he was walking his dog. Worried this time, he had gone to his doctor, who had sent him to the hospital to be investigated. He had been found to have a slight narrowing of one of his coronary arteries, but it had been judged to be too slight to justify surgery.

He came to see me to discover if anything could be done to minimize his chest pain, which was not only a nuisance but also posed a continual threat to him. Apart from the angina, he tired very easily and had troublesome indigestion and mild fibrositis between his shoulders. I found a great deal of spasm in his paravertebral muscles from the neck to the lumbar region. He had treatment to that part of the spine, at the end of which he felt better than he had for years, lost his indigestion and tensed-up state and, after five years, had not had another pain in his chest.

If you have already had a coronary, you should seek this sort of preventative treatment as soon as you have been released from immediate care following the attack and returned to some sort of normality. It is important not to have preventative treatment too soon because it is very tiring. Your body is already working at full stretch to put your heart right, and you don't want to divert energy from this vital task.

# 10 BACK TO GOOD HEALTH

## Treatment for your back problem

Physicians of the utmost fame
Were called at once but when they came
They answered as they took their fees
'There is no cure for this disease.'

Oh, but there is! Some people are sceptical at first but afterwards they marvel at how the treatment has worked where all else failed. This is most rewarding, but I find it hard to share their excitement about the method. Given that the original cause is an old injury, the treatment is so logical that its success is something to be expected.

## ANOTHER LOOK AT THE CAUSE OF BACK PROBLEMS

For a full appreciation of the treatment it is necessary to understand the cause of your non-specific back pain. To recap, an accident, such as a fall from a swing or horse, a skiing or car accident or a hard rugby tackle, gave a jolt to your spine. The blow was largely absorbed by both an increase in the curve of your backbone and also by the elasticity of the discs. The stabilizing joints – the facet joints – not being capable of the same amount of movement as the discs, ultimately took the brunt of the blow and thus became bruised.

There is a mechanism in the body whereby impulses originating in bruised joints travel along the nerves to the spinal cord and then go straight to the muscles across the joint, putting them into a powerful contraction called a spasm. This produces an effect rather like a corset of muscles that is designed to limit movement, thereby giving the joints a rest and speeding recovery. Unfortunately, in the case of the facet joints it is one of nature's bad misfires. In practice, the spasm puts enormous pressure on the facet joints and does very little to limit movement. The joints are not rested and every time they move, the strain is greatly increased.

This sorry state of affairs is greatly aggravated by the fact that an important function of muscles is to return blood to the heart from the tissues. Every time a muscle contracts the tissues tighten both in the muscle and in adjacent areas. This forces fluid out of the tissue spaces into the veins where non-return valves ensure that it makes steady progress back to the heart. As the muscles in a spasm are permanently contracted, this pumping effect is interfered with and leads to excessive fluid, known as oedema, collecting in the area. The build-up of oedema has the effect of diminishing the circulation to the tissues, which not only delays recovery of the damage to the joints but even causes further deterioration. This affects tissues nearby, such as the sympathetic nerve ganglia, causing the related illnesses we discussed earlier.

## TREATING THE BASIC PROBLEM

Clearly, the basis of the problem is largely mechanical. The sufferer has bruised facet joints that have caused a powerful protective spasm of the muscles. Unfortunately, this keeps the problem going. Treatment must promote suitable conditions for the body to heal these damaged joints.

The muscle spasm must be reduced so that some pressure is taken off the joints and the tissue circulation needs to be improved so that the stagnant oedema is squeezed out of the tissue spaces, making room for the fresh fluid to filter in. The ligaments also need to be stretched if relief is to be permanent. When the muscles are in spasm and the discs are compressed for a long period of time these tend to shorten, to take up the slack. Unless they are made to revert to their former length they will continue to exert pressure on the joint surfaces and so interfere with a treatment designed to take the pressure off the facet joints.

The tools that I have found best to achieve this are massage, mobilization, manipulation, ultrasonic waves, surged faradism in the form of a square-wave pulse and the application of cold. I also use drugs as and when indicated – pain-killers, anti-inflammatory drugs and muscle relaxants.

### Over-riding nature's cure

If the facet joints are to be given a chance to recover, the body's own emergency defence repair mechanism must be neutralized to a great extent. Nature's cure for a bruised joint is a protective muscle spasm and an inflammatory process. It is worth looking again at the functions and relationships of the various components of normal circulation.

Consider the tissues as a town in the country, with the houses representing the tissue cells and the streets the tissue spaces. Cars, vans and lorries are the tissue fluids that carry fresh supplies, building materials and workers, i.e. oxygen, sugar and other essentials, into the town (the tissues) and take away the refuse, i.e. carbon dioxide and other waste products.

Now let us suppose that the town is connected to the rest of the country by a railway line (the arteries and veins). When a train, which in this analogy is the blood, stops in the station (the capillaries), the train offloads the cars, vans and lorries from its wagons into the streets of the town. When they have performed their tasks they are reloaded on to the train, now full of waste materials, to be removed. The process is repeated again and again.

An injury could be likened to a fire in a house in the town – the inflammatory reaction would be the attempt to deal with it. Messages go to the fire brigade and cause an over-zealous administration to direct a thousand or so fire engines to the blaze. These are accompanied by a large number of police cars, motorcycles and ambulances. At the same time it is business as usual for the normal population and traffic in the streets. As you can well imagine, this may easily cause a traffic jam that could bring the whole system to a near standstill.

The number of trains increases and extra lines to the station may be opened up but, being unable to unload owing to the already crowded streets, the trains pass straight through the station. In the body, the excessive tissue fluid is such that it actually bulges the tissues, resulting in a local swelling. The inflamed tissues throb with the thunder of the extra blood supply.

People and supplies can no longer get through to the shops and the dustcarts can no longer collect the refuse. If the jam continues for too long, a partial breakdown in the ordinary running and maintenance of the town may result.

This is what happens in the body. Poor circulation in the tissues not only delays recovery of the damage to the joints but also results in further deterioration in them. It also affects nearby tissues such as the sympathetic nerve ganglia.

If it were unable to reach the fire, a wonderful new fire extinguisher would be of limited use to the fire brigade. In the same way, an anti-inflammatory drug is often of limited value if it is unable to reach the tissue concerned. However, if a number of vehicles could be plucked from the streets by helicopters, there would be an immediate improvement in the movement of the cars. This is roughly what ultrasonic waves do to the tissue fluids.

Allowing for a bit of artistic licence, I actually squeeze the town, reducing it to about two-thirds of its original size. This pushes a large number of lorries and cars out of the street back on to the trains to be carried away, thus improving the movement of vehicles in the town and enabling the fire brigade to get through to the fire. This is achieved by making the muscles in the area contract with an electrical impulse – a square-wave pulse – which activates the muscle pump. With the improved circulation, anti-inflammatory drugs can be of great help in speeding up the repair process.

### Surged faradism

Use of this electrical impulse stimulates the nerve that supplies the muscles, making them contract and relax rhythmically at the optimum speed to activate the muscle pump and improve circulation in the area. There is considerable latitude in the surge and rest period. I have found that a three second surge followed by a three second rest works very satisfactorily. This is the most important part of the treatment as the traffic jam of fluid in the tissue spaces is the biggest single factor in delaying recovery.

Patients often comment that they can feel the muscular contraction and relaxation doing good, and although some feel slightly anxious that they have no control over it, the majority say that they know instinctively that this is exactly what their backs need.

Faradic machines are becoming difficult to obtain. Fortunately, all is not lost, as a number of Tens machines have a surge on them and activate the muscle pump perfectly well.

INTERFERENTIAL TREATMENT

This is a form of electrical treatment that is often substituted for surged faradism by physiotherapists. However, it does not activate the muscle pump and is therefore of no use in unclogging the tissue spaces. People given interferential treatment almost always fail to make proper progress.

It is important that faradism is not given at an uncomfortably strong level or carried out for too long. Extra muscular activity greatly increases the arterial blood supply and, as the supply continues for some while after treatment has finished, it would flood out the area again, impeding the tissue circulation and frustrating the whole beneficial effect of the treatment. About three minutes seems to be a good average time for faradism.

This story illustrates the need for moderation.

The matron of my hospital, aged 54, had broken her back a year previously. She was still in a great deal of pain so I was asked to see her. The fracture had healed completely but she was having severe pain in the muscles, which were in a protective spasm from the injury to the facet joints sustained at the time of the fracture.

I instructed the physio superintendent to administer, on alternate days, three minutes of faradism, five minutes of massage, plus 10 minutes of ultrasonic treatment and gentle remobilization. The next week on my return to the hospital everybody gave me black looks.

'I thought your treatment was supposed to make people feel better,' said a doctor. 'We are horrified. It has nearly killed Matron.'

I sought the physio superintendent.

'What have you done to Matron?' I demanded.

'Well, I know you were trying to spare a busy department but as it was Matron I am happy to say that I was able to spare a physio every day. We also upped your almost non-existent treatment to something worthwhile – so we gave half an hour of faradism, half an hour of massage and extensive remobilization.'

It took Matron a fortnight to get over this so that treatment could be resumed. Happily, in the end, she made a good recovery.

Faradism can make things worse if you have a virus infection, and menstruation is sometimes heavier if the electricity is applied in the mid lumbar region, so these can be reasons not to use it for a while. It should also be avoided during the first three months of pregnancy because there may be a slight possibility of it dislodging a precariously implanted ovum in the early stages.

### Remobilization and manipulation

Linchpins of the treatment, these two techniques serve more than one essential purpose.

- **Manipulation can relieve severe pain.** The back is easier to treat when it is symptomless, but unfortunately people tend to come to the doctor only when the pain has become unbearable. So before treating the basic condition, the pain must be eased. The most common pain in the back is due to a muscle in a cramp. Often this is aggravated by the fact that the muscle's long tendon becomes hooked round a bone and remains stretched. This makes it even more painful and prevents it from coming out of the cramp. Manipulation will free the muscle from the bone, often with a loud click, enabling it to shorten and quickly come out of the cramp.

- **Manipulation can also free a nerve that is pinched in a neural canal.** This occurs when the facet joint – which, as figure 4.2 on page 75 shows, forms part of the canal – swells into the canal and thus pinches the nerve. Manipulation can open up the joint and so lift the pressure off the nerve, lessening the pain almost instantaneously.

- **Remobilization has a vital part to play in ensuring reasonably permanent relief**. When a muscle is in spasm the vertebrae are pulled together, compressing the elastic intervertebral discs. After a while, the ligaments contract to take up the slack. So, even when the muscle spasm is relaxed, there is little improvement as the shortened ligaments continue to exert considerable pressure on the facet joints. Repeated, gentle remobilization can stretch the ligaments back to the right length and help keep the muscle from going back into spasm.

- **Remobilization can be used to treat neural tethering.** The sheath of the nerves may become fixed at the base of the skull or where the nerve roots pass through the neural canals at the low lumbar or sacral sections of the spinal column. As an example of how remobilization exercises can help, if this affects a leg, sit on a couch with your legs stretched out straight in front and slump forward as far as possible. Your practitioner should, gently but firmly, push your head down while lifting the affected leg as high as you allow. This can be repeated several times. An exercise to do at home in between treatments is to stand with the affected leg propped on a stool. Bend forward, putting your weight on to the leg and forcing your body down over it.

### Firm but gentle massage

This both encourages the muscle to come out of spasm and squeezes the oedema out of the affected area into the veins, helping to normalize the circulation to some extent. The intensity of massage must be carefully calculated – firm enough to produce the desired effects but not so vigorous or prolonged as to stimulate an increased the arterial supply (because this will flood the area later, as in the case of too much faradism). Rub the back of your hand vigorously for a while and it will begin to go red due to the increased arterial circulation. Excessive massage has the same effect deeper in the tissues.

### Power-assisted micro-manipulation (PAM)

The machine that administers this very useful treatment has 'fingers' that fit over the transverse processes of two adjacent vertebrae and twists them in opposite directions. It is able to perform rapid controlled manipulations that would be very difficult to emulate by hand. The treatment is very good for sorting out abnormal curves of the spine, including a scoliosis, which is a lateral curvature.

### Ultrasonic waves

The most dispensable tools of the treatment, patients will almost always improve without the use of these sound waves, but recovery will take longer. Ultrasonic waves hit a far higher note than a human, or even a dog, can hear. With good hearing, you can hear about 17,000 vibrations a second; the frequency I use is three million vibrations a second (3MHz).

Ultrasonic waves help in several ways

- When waves of above two watts to the square centimetre (a very weak dose) are applied to the muscles that are in spasm, they have the effect of contracting the arterioles, which lessens the supply of blood to the area and helps to get rid of the jam. On average, I use about two and a half watts to the square centimetre, which is still a very small dose. In the early days we used to go up to 100 watts, but this was often very uncomfortable and even painful for the patient. The dose was gradually reduced until we reached the present level of two and a half watts or below, according to where the treatment is being used. A lower intensity tends to open up arterioles thus increasing the arterial supply. This, of course, frustrates the thrust of the treatment in reducing tissue fluids. Therapeutically, these small doses are just as effective as the higher ones.

- Ultrasonic waves speed up chemical reactions, probably by buffeting molecules about so they meet each other more frequently. This, of course, makes the healing processes much faster.
- They may also alter the filtration pressure of the tissue fluid by making some of the big protein molecules stick together, thereby increasing the filtration pressure of the tissue fluid. This causes the fluid to be drawn out of the area, back into the blood vessels by a force known as osmosis.
- Ultrasonic waves applied directly over the facet joints encourage muscles to come out of a cramp or spasm and this greatly speeds up the repair processes. Patients find it soothing and most say they can actually feel the improvement.

A more effective treatment is the longer wave ultrasonic with a cone-shaped output. This penetrates deeper and goes more effectively into joints as the wave travels in so many different directions. The machine is called a Physassist.

Drugs

Those used in the treatment of back trouble are mainly analgesics, anti-inflammatory drugs and muscle relaxants.

- **Analgesics** are simply pain relievers. The most effective, including aspirin, are mild with the advantage of being anti-inflammatory as well. The disadvantage is that they can cause bleeding in the stomach – and, very rarely, an allergic reaction.

  – *Paracetamol* is similar to aspirin in strength and does not upset the stomach – but neither does it have any anti-inflammatory effect. It is very safe but can damage the liver if taken in excess. Liver patients should not take paracetamol.
  – *Co-proxamol* (better known as distalgesic) is a more powerful pain reliever, does not upset the stomach but also has no anti-inflammatory effect.
  – *Dihydrocodeine (DF118)* is a much more powerful drug and it can sometimes make you feel a little peculiar or nauseous. It is effective, however, when the pain is extremely severe.
  – *Morphine, phenazocine and methadone* are all very powerful pain relievers and should be used with great caution – maybe to alleviate acute pain until the attack is on the wane. The more powerful drugs can be obtained by prescription only.

- **Anti-inflammatory drugs** are a large group that work by preventing the production of the prostaglandins that stimulate the inflammatory reaction. This reaction may be the mechanism of repair but if the inflammation becomes excessive, it can markedly interfere with recovery. Reducing it can thus aid the recovery process. These drugs fall into two main groups:

– *Steroids* are very potent but are prone to cause side-effects if given over a prolonged period. Tablets given in a relatively large dose over a period of a month or two can sometimes lead to a breakthrough in an unusually stubborn condition.

Injections of cortisone, the best-known substance in this group, are something of a mixed blessing. The cortisone can be injected directly – often combined with an analgesic – into tender trigger spots, or into or around the facet joints. In this case, the needle goes into the space between the spinal cord complex and the bones of the spinal canal (an epidural injection). This enables the cortisone to travel some distance without any risk to the spinal cord itself, and to bathe the nerve roots and facet joints. The cortisone reduces the inflammation of the facet joints resulting in a lessening of the spasm. It is often administered for referred pain in a leg.

If you make a good recovery while the cortisone is active, you may well have prolonged relief from pain. Unfortunately, for some people these injections can cause deterioration of the joints, which leaves them in a considerably worse state. Subsequent injections seldom seem to help as much as the original one.

– *Non-steroidal anti-inflammatory drugs (NSAIDs)* are not so effective but on the whole much safer than steroids. They work by inhibiting the Cox enzymes that help to produce the prostaglandins. Unfortunately, one type of prostaglandin helps to protect the stomach and is produced by the Cox 1 enzyme. Most of the NSAIDs affect both Cox 1 and 2 enzymes. Recently, however, new drugs that affect the Cox 2 enzyme only, such as Vioxx, have become available, and are much less likely to affect the stomach.

People react differently to different preparations, so it is usually worth changing to another brand if the first one doesn't work very well or doesn't agree with you. Many of them work much more efficiently if administered in the form of a suppository. Examples of these drugs are Brufen, Feldene, Froben, Indocid, Naprosyn, Ponstan and Voltarol. Most require a prescription from your doctor.

■ **Muscle relaxants** work through the brain to relax the muscle spasm. They can be helpful for people who have had back trouble for years and are difficult to treat, and for those who are tense and rigid during manipulation.

Probably the most commonly used is diazepam (Valium), which is very effective. I am not in favour of using this drug because it is addictive and patients can have difficulty discontinuing its use even after a comparatively short course.

A much safer, and effective, alternative is to take a small daily dose – 10 to 20 milligrams – of amitrityline. In this dosage, amitrityline is virtually just a muscle relaxant although it may make you feel a little spaced out for the first day or two. Very rarely, it does not suit someone and, in this case, will make you feel very peculiar. Diazepam or another antidepressant is the alternative, and it may be better to rely on pain-killers and anti-inflammatory drugs.

MINERAL DEFICIENCY

Lack of calcium, magnesium and occasionally sodium (common salt) causes muscles to go into a cramp. A shortage of the first two usually causes cramps in the feet or calf muscles at night. Taking supplements will rapidly restore the electrolyte balance and stop the cramps. These deficiencies can make the back muscles almost as sensitive as the legs, causing or maintaining back pain. Calcium is far and away the most common deficiency.

■ **The application of cold** to the relevant part of the body with an ice-pack, a spray or a pack of frozen peas – petits pois are best because they mould so well to the body – closes down the arterial circulation in that area. The body's natural reaction is to conserve heat by not allowing too much blood to become cooled.

This effect lasts quite a long time after the source of the cold has been removed. As a result of the reduction in the arterial blood supply, less fluid enters the tissue spaces to replace the fluid that has diffused out. Therefore the tissue-fluid pressure lessens and more fluid is able to flow through the tissue spaces.

Cold also reduces the sensitivity of the nerves – remember the snake that could hardly move when cold? This means that the impulses that would have been transmitted to the muscles from the bruised area are greatly diminished and the protective spasm is reduced proportionately. The easing of pressure on the facet joints, together with the slight improvement in the muscle pump, helps to speed up recovery.

Another effect of a decrease in the nerve impulses is to lessen the sensation of pain, sometimes quite dramatically.

## SOME QUESTIONS ANSWERED

*How long does the treatment take to work?*

This is a difficult question to answer because, as the case histories cited illustrate, there are considerable variations in the basic problem and thus the time it takes to regain a healthy back. Also, similar people with similar complaints can take widely differing times to recover. The average seems to be around six to twelve visits but some people need fewer sessions, some need many more.

For the treatment to be successful, it is essential to see it through to the end. It is rather like pushing a sledge up a snowy slope. If you leave it 10 feet from the top and go home for dinner, it will have slipped some distance down the slope by the time you get back. If you push it right to the top before you leave, it is far more likely to stay there.

The measure of recovery is the degree of spasm in the muscles, which can be felt by palpation. The end of the spasm can be quite difficult to feel, so it is always hard to know exactly when there has been a full recovery. It is for this reason that I ask patients to come back after three months for a further check to see if any more treatment is required – but once it has gone, it is unlikely that the original spasm will return.

After the first treatment, there is a marked improvement in the conditions needed for the repair of the facet joints – the muscles are more relaxed and the stale oedema has been pumped out of the tissue spaces in favour of refreshed fluid. The joints will begin to heal and the spasm will begin to become less intense.

However, after a day or so, when the repair has improved the situation about 10 to 20 per cent, the body mechanism puts the muscles back into spasm, thus halting the repair. By the time the patient comes back for the second treatment, the spasm is usually around 10 per cent better. After this and subsequent treatments, the same happens except that the benefit may last longer.

As the joints improve, there is a corresponding reduction in the number of impulses travelling from the damaged areas to the muscles, telling them to contract, so the degree of spasm is roughly proportional to the level of trouble in the joints.

*I've had back trouble for 20 years. Have I left it too late for treatment?*

Given the right conditions, the body is just as capable of repairing the facet joints after 15 or 20 years as it is after a month. The bruised facet joints and the muscle spasm reach a relatively stable state early on and this rarely alters much over the years. The spasm may very slowly cause the bruising to increase but, in general, something of a status quo is established. There is no built-in clock and the body is unaware of how long the problem has been present.

*Does the treatment hurt?*

This is a common concern and, fortunately, the answer is no. Indeed, many people find it very relaxing. Of course, there may be the occasional momentary twinge, but the principle of the treatment is that it must not hurt. It is important to remember that the treatment is only trying to put the repair mechanism into order so that the body can heal itself. On its own, it cannot actually repair anything. Pain is the ultimate alarm bell informing the body that something is wrong. If treatment hurts, the body will resist, eventually blocking any beneficial effect.

*How will I feel afterwards?*

After each treatment, the amount of pain suffered depends on what you do. Going on a car journey, for instance, or taking part in any other activity likely to cause back pain may not be a good idea. Feeling anxious doesn't help and even food, drink and the weather can have an effect. Good days and bad days are not a measure of the real state of progress. The degree of spasm being generated by the inflammation in the joints is the only true indication of improvement.

The first one or two treatments are usually given very gently as they can be extremely fatiguing, especially for those with upper-back problems. Most feel very tired for some hours afterwards, or even all of the next day. This is because the treatment tends to upset the sympathetic nervous system, which is already in disarray, and as it has not yet had time to make any marked improvement, the system may actually malfunction even more.

Some people, fortunately few in numbers, are made worse by the treatment for a short while. Massage, for example, involves rubbing cells together, and if these are badly injured they may not respond well. The overall effect of the treatment is vastly more beneficial than harmful but can produce a mild reaction, especially in the early stages before much improvement has taken place. This applies especially to migraine sufferers.

If you feel that you are not much better after several weeks, this may simply be because, having felt some improvement, you are now more sensitive to pain. Remember, your pain threshold varies according to circumstances, and your awareness increases considerably after a rest from the stimulus. Go into the fresh air from a room with a bad smell, or into the cold after time spent in a hot atmosphere, and then go back inside, and the smell or the heat seem many times worse. In the same way, you can get so used to pain after a while that your body becomes less sensitive to it but, given a period of improvement, the same level of pain will seem considerably enhanced.

After a few pain-free weeks, you may suddenly have a bad day. In fact, the final twinges may not stop until two or three months after the last treatment as the arterial circulation generated by the repair mechanism can still flood the muscles and cause a cramp but, with the bruising recovered, this circulation gradually returns to normal.

*My mother is 80 – is she too old for treatment?*

It is one of the saddest misconceptions that people become too old to have successful treatment. Indeed, the young and very strong are often the most difficult to treat. As we have seen, the main enemy of the painful back is an over-enthusiastic repair mechanism. People over the age of 65 or 70 almost certainly have a good repair mechanism to have survived so long. The adverse effects of a muscle spasm greatly diminish with age and so oppose the treatment far less. On the whole, older people respond to treatment more quickly than their younger counterparts.

*Where can I get this treatment?*

Most physiotherapists have the necessary equipment and knowledge to give the treatment. All it requires is a minor modification of methods that are already in use. Your doctor will almost certainly be able to recommend someone who can offer surged faradism and possibly ultrasonic waves. The physiotherapist should be well versed in remobilization techniques.

Some osteopaths and chiropractors also have the necessary skills of manipulation, and use the same equipment, and they will be able to give the treatment equally efficiently. A detailed description of the treatment is given in Appendix I, page 249.

## OTHER AVAILABLE TREATMENTS

### Abraham's box
This treatment is based on radionics and the belief that all substances, and human beings, emit radiation. The theory is that if something goes wrong in the body, the ray from an offending tissue is altered. The

box detects this and gives out a correcting ray, which will cure the patient.

### Acupressure or shiatsu

Direct pressure is applied with a finger or knuckle to acupuncture and other tender points, often followed by a general massage. Derived from acupuncture over the last 45 years, the effect is not as good as that obtained by using needles. Originally, it was used for relief of fatigue and as a general tone-up. More recently, however, it has been employed both to diagnose and treat conditions similar to those treated by acupuncture.

### Acupuncture

This technique originated in Ancient China and it remains one of the mainstays of Chinese medical practice. Widely adopted in Western cultures, it has many advocates. Some practitioners use the old Chinese theory of balancing rival forces in the body, the imbalance of which has brought about a particular disease, by implanting needles in a choice of sites. This has several medically understandable effects.

- When the skin is punctured the body secretes powerful analgesics called endorphins that tend to block the passage of pain impulses.
- Sensory impulses from the skin will, to a varying degree, block the passage of impulses up the pain-carrying nerves associated with this area. This is the same principle that you have probably noticed when you have a painful spot and either press on it or rub it hard and the pain is greatly alleviated. This is also the basis of TENS (transcutaneous electrical nerve stimulation, see page 236).
- The fight-or-flight mechanism will kick in if there is a perceived external threat, such as a lion standing 100 yards away. Internal

pain, such as an ache in the back or knee, will be counteracted. Puncturing the skin could be the ultimate threat and so bring about a marked relief from the pain.

– A barrage of impulses from a trigger point sends impulses to the associated muscles causing a correcting redistribution of chemicals in the fibres, resulting in the muscle relaxing from a cramp. This would, of course, relieve the pain, and by taking some of the pressure off the facet joint in the back, the conditions for this to repair itself would become much more favourable.

– With some practitioners there may be an element of hypnotism brought about by the accompanying reassurance and constant suggestion that the condition is improving.

Acupuncture does seem to work for many people, although the benefits may be short-term.

Modern versions of the technique in widespread use include passing electrical impulses through the needles to enhance the effect. This is called electro-acupuncture.

Another variation is to heat the trigger spot with a herb called Moxa. As soon as the glowing bundle of the herb makes the skin feel hot, it is removed. A smouldering Moxa stick may be held near each trigger point to achieve the same effect. The Moxa may also be burned on the top of the acupuncture needle so that the heat is transmitted down it.

A recent variation of the acupuncture principle of pain-blocking by stimulating the skin is transcutaneous electrical nerve stimulation (TENS). Small electrical pads spaced over the trigger points are stimulated with a battery operated by a low-frequency current. This can give considerable relief, even with severe pain, and can be used at home or anywhere. Women in childbirth very often use it.

## Alexander technique

Fredrick Alexander, an actor, developed this technique about one hundred years ago in Austria. His chin projected forward more than normal and he found that his voice problems improved when he corrected this postural fault. From this, he went on to form a theory that the original good posture and normal behaviour pattern we display as children is gradually eroded as we develop bad habits in the use of our bodies. These interfere with the proper function of the muscles and nervous system, and result in poor co-ordination and balance. Common faults are tensing muscles, crossing the legs, jutting the chin forward and increasing the curves of the spine.

Treatment involves extensive retraining to correct the faults and it is the considerable commitment of time and effort that is the main drawback in an otherwise excellent and helpful system.

## Aromatherapy

Essential oils derived from a variety of natural sources, such as flowers, seeds, leaves, roots and barks, are the bases of this treatment. Each oil relieves a particular complaint and a mixture is concocted depending on the symptoms. The oils may be administered in several different ways, the most popular being combined with an overall massage or in the form of an inhalation. Many clinics put the oils into a therapeutic hot bath. Recently, a steam aromatherapy tube has been used, which is large enough to allow you to be completely immersed in the aromatic steam.

The oils are very expensive because a great deal of effort is needed to collect all the constituents and to extract the essential substances. Neroli, for example, is drawn from orange blossom petals, and pounds of petals are required to produce one ounce of oil. Fortunately, only very few drops are needed to make up an individual mixture. The oils are very potent and can be dangerous if taken internally. They should be obtained from a reputable dealer only.

Oils that are helpful for back trouble are lavender (in the form of a massage), marjoram and rosemary. Black pepper and ginger are helpful when there is acute pain.

### Bed rest

A sufferer is put to bed and told to stay there until the pain has improved. However, as we have seen in previous chapters, this is not a satisfactory long-term treatment. The lack of activity greatly impairs the circulation, which delays the recovery of the facet joints. Even if the immediate pain is eventually relieved after a period of bed rest, further attacks are usually forthcoming as nothing has been done to correct the basic problem.

### Clinical nutrition

Also referred to as dietary therapy, this focuses on the belief that impurities in the system, mainly derived from processed and nutritionally empty foods, cause arthritic conditions and back pain. The problem is dealt with by eliminating all these processed foods from the diet and following a cleansing regime. Supplementary vitamins and trace elements augment the diet, in particular magnesium, calcium and potassium.

### Corsets, collars and plaster-casts

The main idea is to rest the back. There are certain occasions when this is the best form of treatment because these devices take a great deal of the load off the muscles, thus reducing their requirements of oxygen and food from the limited circulation that is available and offering temporary relief. One major benefit of wearing a corset or collar is the support it offers while standing or during a car journey. In general, they have the same disadvantages as bed rest.

Plaster-casts are a drastic version of corsets, used as a more complete support for the spine in extreme cases. They are heavy, hot in warmer weather, and also make the wearer clumsy and partly immobile. They usually have to be worn for a few months, and then can be replaced by a corset.

### Exercise

Although exercise plays a vital role in diminishing the symptoms of back trouble, as I pointed out in chapter 4, I do seriously question whether it is of any help in correcting the basic problem. Once you stop, the pain will return, and I see many patients who exercise regularly as instructed and still have back pain.

Aerobics involve many different pumping movements of the arms and legs, but aquarobics and aquacise (aqua-exercise) are preferable because some of the unacceptable strain on the back is removed. Swimming is good exercise as long as the strokes are varied. Holding the head up for a long time while swimming the breaststroke puts a considerable strain on the neck.

### Faith, spiritual and natural healing

Power is said to pass from the healer to the patient so that the patient's own mechanism heals the body. The source of power varies with the healer. Faith healers believe in using the patient's own religious beliefs to motivate healing. Others believe that they channel a 'divine force' or are directed by a spiritual guide. Hostile influences, such as anger, are eliminated and the patient acquires a changed state of mind. There is no explanation of what really happens but many cases of cures have been documented. Unfortunately, this kind of healing is open to quackery so some caution is needed in the choice of therapist.

## Homoeopathy

Samuel Hahnemann originated this therapy in Germany towards the end of the sixteenth century. The orthodox treatments of the day were blood-letting, drastic purges – which had much the same effect as dysentery – and large doses of often toxic drugs. It has been estimated that the average mortality rate from the treatments alone was in excess of 20 per cent. If the patient had no treatment at all, the chances of survival were that much greater.

Hahnemann thought that taking substances that produced the symptoms of the disease in very small quantities would provoke the body's own repair mechanism, provided medicines were not be mixed. Towards the end of his life he put forward the idea that the more diluted the solution of the medicine, the greater the potency or effect.

It is difficult to produce pain in the back with any medicine so homoeopathy is not an obvious choice of treatment, but several of my patients have taken homoeopathic anti-inflammatory drugs, which have proved most effective. There are specific homoeopathic remedies for lumbago, coccyalgia (pain around the coccyx), prolapsed discs, fibrositis, Paget's disease and ankylosing spondylitis.

## Hydrotherapy

The ancient baths found all over Europe testify to the popularity of this therapy in Greek and Roman days. It can be beneficial from the point of view of the exercise that can be taken in the weightless environment of water, and because various minerals – either occurring naturally or subsequently added – are absorbed through the skin. In a number of spas, the water may be drunk.

There are many variations of the treatment. Jets can be used to stimulate the skin. The water may be hot or cold – patients may alternate from one to the other. Sitz baths employ this technique and are very popular in health clinics.

### Injections of sclerosing agents

This involves injecting a substance to irritate the tissues, such as a strong sugar solution, resulting in the production of fibrous tissue, which is designed to stiffen or stabilize the painful part of the back. These injections – a form of built-in corset – are very effective for some people but if they are not successful, you may be even worse than before and the back problems can be more difficult to treat by other means.

### Manipulation and remobilization

These tools are used by various disciplines and, as already noted, I use them myself. Remobilization is a gentle encouragement of movement of joints and tissues, whereas manipulation is a forceful thrust in the desired direction beyond the previously possible range of movement. Orthopaedic manipulation is a rather drastic way of trying to solve the problem. It is often given under anaesthetic and tends to be of a rather violent nature.

Massage is the medical term for manipulation of the soft tissues and this can take many forms.

### PRACTITIONERS

Many physiotherapists use the techniques of remobilization and manipulation to a very high standard. There are several methods but I prefer the Maitland system because it is gentle and nearest to my own technique. Maitland, an Australian physiotherapist, wrote a book describing manipulative and remobilizing techniques that some regard as the physiotherapist's bible.

Apart from massage, other means employed by physiotherapists include hot wax, hot and cold treatment, baths, short-waves or microwaves, laser treatment and exercises. They often achieve very good results treating an attack of back pain.

Bone-setting – an intuitive manipulative treatment popular all over America in the nineteenth century – was developed into osteopathy by Andrew Still in 1874. He postulated that any interference with the nerve or blood supply to the tissues as a result of a structural problem, such as a curvature or muscle spasm in the spine, would prevent normal healing taking place. Treatment was to realign the structural and soft tissue problems that could cause the interference.

Later, in about 1895, D.D. Palmer developed another technique from the practices of the American bone-setters. Chiropractic involves rectifying misalignments of the bones of the spine and other parts of the body to alleviate disturbances of the nervous system caused by them. Chiropractors do not use drugs.

The manipulation used in naturopathy is similar to, or the same as, that used in osteopathy. The system goes further, though, involving reinforcing the body's natural defences by fasting and diet, hydrotherapy, removal of physical tension to release psychological causes of illness, acupuncture, herbalism and homoeopathy.

I believe that both osteopaths and chiropractors are giving the correct treatment for back problems, but possibly for the wrong reason. Both methods of manipulation have the basic aim of putting back displaced vertebrae. However, as figure 10.1 shows, the vertebrae are locked together most effectively. Indeed, it is hard to see how vertebrae can be displaced, and if they are not displaced, there is no displacement to rectify.

Suitable manipulation by osteopaths and chiropractors does relieve back pain but this is not because it puts back a displaced vertebra. As discussed in chapter 4, the click so often heard is, in fact, the freeing of a muscle tendon that has become hooked around a bony projection. The moment the muscle is able to shorten, which is what occurs when my prescribed treatment is undertaken, it starts to come out of cramp and the pain stops.

This kind of manipulation offers relief but it does not help the underlying problem. Nothing has been done to repair the bruised facet joints, so the muscles nearly always return to their original spasm and, in most cases, manipulation is needed again. Each manipulation will ease the pain of individual attacks but as conditions in the muscle

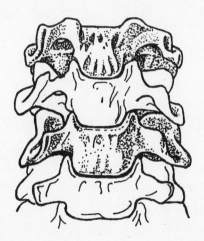

Figure 10.1 The strong, close-fitting and interlocking structure of the vertebrae makes displacement extremely difficult.

deteriorate, it becomes easier and easier to put it into a cramp. When reasonably normal, something as drastic as lifting a sideboard would be needed to set it off. Later, just leaning forward could do it and there comes a time when a muscle will go into cramp even though it is not being stretched. It is at this point that manipulation can no longer relieve the pain, as the muscle is not trapped. It cannot be helped by attempting to shorten it, for it is already of normal length. It is at this point that patients tend to come to me.

### Medical herbalism

One of the oldest forms of medical treatment, this has its roots in Ancient China. The main conflict between medical herbalists and doctors lies in the belief of the herbalist that the potency of the active ingredient is diminished both by purifying it and by the loss of other substances in the herb that, when present, enhance its action. They also believe that synthetic copies are less effective.

Doctors, on the other hand, are convinced that it is enormously preferable to have a substance the exact effect of which is known and which, as it is pure, can be put into measured quantities, ensuring that the patient receives a totally predictable dose. It has been found, for instance, that the amount of active ingredient in a foxglove leaf (Digitalis purpurea) varies from one plant to another. A heart patient being treated by the leaf might receive either a serious overdose or one just sufficient to help the condition.

Herbalists treat the whole body in correcting a complaint. Back pain is not really one of their strong points but the treatment may help. For instance, the application of silver birch bark may ease tender muscles, and a poultice of mustard seed relieves skeletal pain. An infusion of valerian, taken internally, relieves pain. Remember that some herbs may be dangerous. Consult a registered herbalist.

## Meditation

Apart from any of the other benefits this may provide, it does help to ease back pain by relaxing the muscles. Their tightness makes an attack of pain more likely and inhibits the mechanism of repair. Meditation can be very helpful in both respects.

## Reflexology

The Egyptians, among other ancient peoples, believed that the body is divided into 10 zones that are represented by different areas on the toes and fingers. Around 1930, an American masseuse, Eunice Ingham, drew up a map showing where on the feet the reflex zones affected by various parts of the body are located. Treatment consists of deep massage of the relevant areas of the feet, said to be particularly helpful with neck, shoulder and back pain.

## Surgery

In my view, surgery should be restricted to the small minority of cases where there is a mechanical defect. This may be a ruptured disc, a vertebra that has slipped or a very unstable relationship between two vertebrae. The first needs removal, the other two need stabilizing by means of a bone graft or some other mechanical device.

## Traction

This is something of a double-edged sword. The advantages are that while the muscle is in traction, the joints are freed from the pressure of the spasm and have the opportunity to repair themselves. However, the muscle pump often becomes even more inefficient and so the joints do not always repair effectively. The muscles may also react badly to being stretched and go into a powerful and painful cramp once the traction is released. Some problems are helped by traction, others are made markedly worse.

## Yoga

Designed to increase the life force in the body, I strongly recommend this excellent Indian system to back-pain sufferers. As in most exercise routines, there are a few movements that may stress the back and exacerbate the pain but these will become obvious fairly rapidly and can be avoided. A yoga teacher will be able to offer advice about the best routine to follow. Mantra, or nada, yoga is probably the best for pain relief as it affects the endocrine system.

## AIDS TO REDUCE BACK STRAIN

There are many forms of artificial aid to reduce strain on the back. The following are some of the most basic.

- **Beds.** We spend a large proportion of our lives in bed so, when buying one, it is worth spending as much money as you can reasonably afford. Choose one made by a reputable manufacturer. Mattresses may be expensive because of the cost of the coverings rather than because they better in the spring department. A good salesman will be able to compare the supportive qualities of various ranges. Orthopaedic beds are usually too hard and, although better than a soft sagging mattress, may not give as restful a night as a firm grade of a reputable make.

### THE START OF ORTHOPAEDICS

The word orthopaedic has an interesting history. Orthos means straight and paidos means a child. The word derives from the time when many children had tubercular vertebrae. These would eventually collapse, leaving the child a hunchback or, at the very least, with a horribly distorted spine. A Welsh blacksmith called Thomas welded the children into an iron support that kept them straight for the year or so that was needed for the spine to heal. When they were released, their backs were straight. His son qualified as a doctor and continued as a child straightener. The medical profession likes everything to be given a Greek or Latin name so he became known as an orthopaedic doctor.

- **Loss of weight.** Even though being overweight is almost certainly not the cause of back trouble, it has some effect on producing back pain. Imagine the extra work your back has to cope with, and without any increase of movement to keep the circulation going. A sensible weight-loss diet is some help in relieving back strain.

- **Massage rollers and vibrating pads**. Wooden rollers used to massage the back can squeeze fluid out of an affected area and improve the basic condition. Vibrating pads and cushions also soothe the back and in moderation can do no harm.

- **Seat lumbar supports.** The muscles are stretched when sitting down and, for the majority of back-pain sufferers, this increases the tendency for them to cramp. A support that pushes the lumbar spine straight can go a long way towards preventing this. Motoring is one of the most trying conditions for a back-pain sufferer, so a lumbar support is even more beneficial in a car.

People with stiff or painful necks can be helped, especially when driving but also sometimes when asleep. Prolonged sitting can make the neck very uncomfortable, so again a support may help.

Chairs are often designed more for appearance than for proper support. Well-designed chairs are an enormous aid to comfort. Choose one that supports the lumbar region.

■ **Shoes.** Special shoes can be helpful for correcting a variety of foot and leg problems. The shoe can be built up to correct a short leg; wedges can be put on the side to correct a tilt of the foot; bars can be placed across the foot to redistribute the weight better. The improved posture can help back pain a great deal. Cushions in the sole of the shoe lessen the jolting effect of walking or running on hard, man-made surfaces, which eases the load on the facet joints and lessens the spasm.

■ **Working surfaces.** Where possible these should be adjusted so that, when standing, bending forward is kept to a minimum. When sitting, you should be able to sit up reasonably straight and keep the arms and hands at a comfortable height.

# APPENDIX

## Description of treatment
## A note for your therapist

The apparatus required is a surged faradic machine (preferably as a square-wave pulse) and an ultrasonic wave generator – any frequency will do but I have found the Physassist the most satisfactory.

There is no particular order in which to give the treatment but it may be preferable to use the machines first if the patient is in a great deal of pain as it soothes the tissues and often relaxes some of the muscle spasm. If, however, there is no severe pain, the patient may find the electrical treatment relaxing after the remobilization or manipulation.

## SURGED FARADISM

The surge needs to be set at a cycle of about three seconds surge and three seconds rest. Extremely rarely, this may provoke a reaction. I use pads about 25cm long and 5cm wide placed on either side of the vertebrae to activate the groups of muscles involved. They may have to be moved and the surge repeated to cover the whole area. The intensity should be turned up gradually until it verges on being uncomfortable, and then eased back a fraction. It is very important that the treatment is completely pain-free and comfortable. If the strength is excessive it will induce an increased blood supply which will continue after the treatment is over. As a result, instead of the tissue fluids being reduced so that there is a better tissue-fluid exchange, the extra circulation will flood the area, defeating the object of the treatment.

## ULTRASONIC WAVES – PULSED

The timing is at the discretion of the operator. Ten minutes over a moderately sized area – half the back or one hip joint – seems a good average. I use from two to five watts per square centimetre as this tends to reduce the arteriole circulation and has a maximal effect on the cramp, spasm and inflamed joint.

I also use it on any secondary site of inflammation, such as the knee, hip or shoulder joint.

## REMOBILIZATION AND MANIPULATION

This is applied to the back and, if suitable, to any secondary site. A Grade V manoeuvre (manipulation) may be necessary but the strength required should first be carefully assessed by test moves.

I use most of the following manoeuvres on the back:

1. Place the left hand flat on the back with the first joint of the thumb just below the vertebral spine, comfortably cradling it. Place the right hand over the left thumb so it fits comfortably between the thenar and hypothenar eminences. Press to take up any slack and then, using the arm and shoulder, push down to give a firm, sharp, downward and horizontal thrust. All vertebrae should be treated in the area of the muscle spasm at Grades IV to V, but tender vertebrae, or those suspected of being at the centre of the referred pain, should receive up to Grade V.

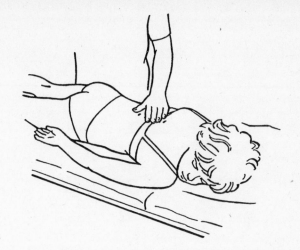

*Figure A1.1*

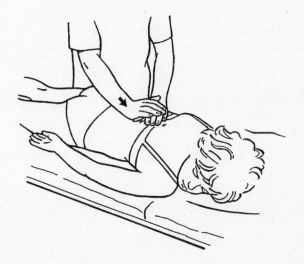

*Figure A1.2*

2. With pain in the low lumbar region, lift up the pelvis by putting the
   right hand under the iliac crest, and lift it about 10cm. Place the ball
   of the left thumb on the other side of the low lumbar vertebral

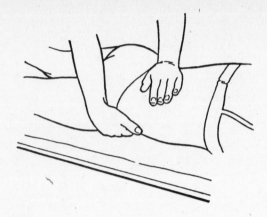

*Figure A1.3*

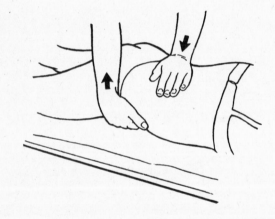

*Figure A1.4*

spine. Give a sharp thrust down with the left hand and a little pull up with the right.

Stand on the other side of the patient and repeat the process.

3. Place the patient on the opposite side to the known pain, the top leg in front and the top shoulder back. Pull the underarm as far forwards as is convenient. Place the left hand on the shoulder and

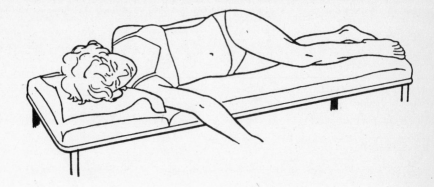

*Figure A1.5*

the other arm on the pelvic crest. Ease the patient as far as he/she can be rotated when relaxed. Take up the strain and give a moderate thrust in the same direction. Repeat the other way with the patient on the painful side but this time use a Grade V thrust.

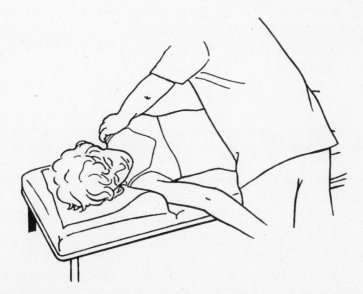

*Figure A1.6*

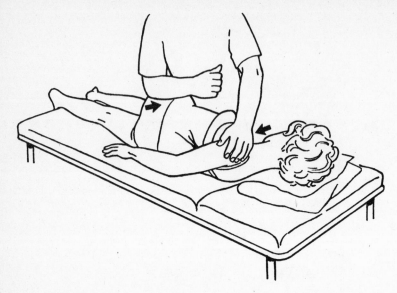

*Figure A1.7*

It is rare for the sharp thrust to be needed the first way – the patient feels the second one more.

If the pain is central, test each way. One way will probably be slightly more uncomfortable than the other. The comfortable side is the one to receive the Grade V thrust.

4. With the patient lying on his/her back and the couch head lifted, cup the chin with one hand and the occiput with the other. Make sure the teeth are closed and the tongue well clear and rotate the head in either direction. One way is almost always more comfortable than the other.

Rotate the head in the less comfortable direction, using considerable traction at the same time. Take up slack – ask the patient to relax as much as possible and to breathe right out. Using the arms and shoulders, give a combined rotatory thrust and pull about Grade IV. Repeat in the other direction, but this time Grade V.

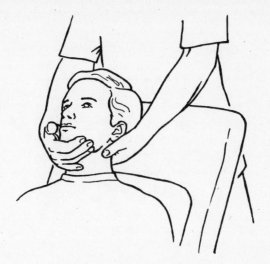

*Figure A1.8*

5. The patient should lie on his/her back on the flat couch with arms crossed and hands grasping opposite shoulders.

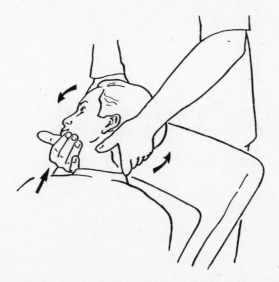

*Figure A1.9*

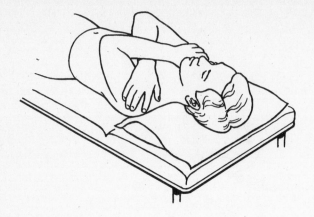

*Figure A1.10*

Stand roughly level with the middle of the chest and lift the far shoulder with your outer arm. Make a fist with your other hand and place it on the back with a vertebral body between the thumb and first finger.

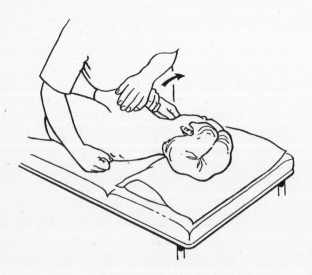

*Figure A1.11*

Rest the patient back flat on to the hand and bend over leaning your chest on the folded elbows. Press through the elbows and chest to the vertebrae and on to the hand to take up all slack. As the patient breathes right out give a sharp thrust through the elbows and chest.

Repeat this throughout the area of muscle spasm. I vary from Grade III in the peripheral areas to Grade V where the back or spine is painful.

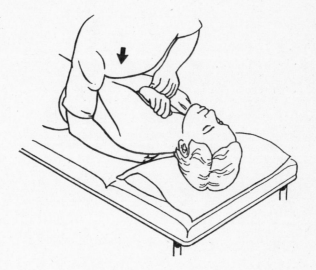

*Figure A1.12*

6. The patient sits on the couch with legs over one side and buttocks well back. He/she grasps both hands behind the neck, or if more comfortable, places the hands just on the base of the neck.

Thread your arms through the patient's arms and grasp the wrists firmly. The patient must lean back and become as limp as possible. Pull the patient's shoulders back and, at the same time, push the chest forward using the abdomen with a small sausage shaped

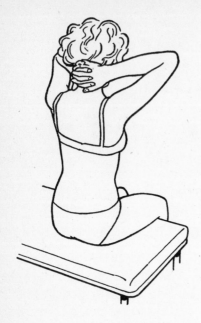

*Figure A1.13*

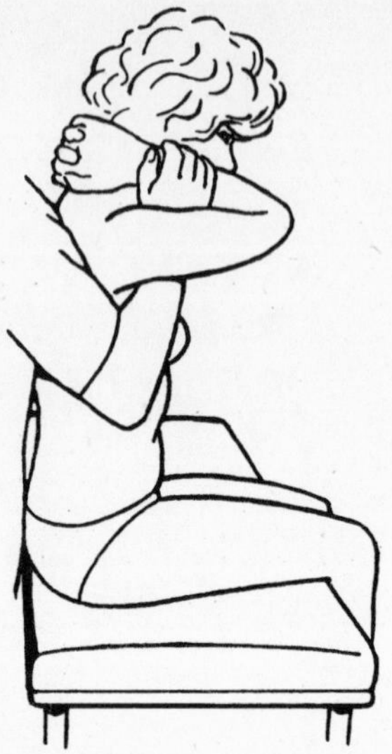

*Figure A1.14*

cushion, loosening the upper thoracic spine.

Repeat the same manoeuvre but this time, when the patient is completely relaxed, give a sharp shrug of the shoulders lifting the patient sharply in an upward direction.

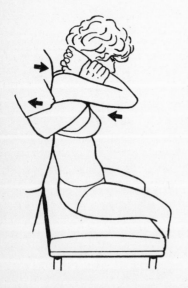

*Figure A1.15*

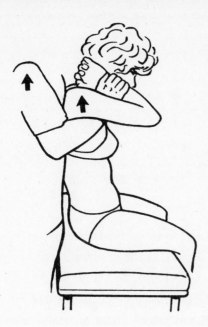

*Figure A1.16*

7. Stand behind the patient, who is sitting on a stool. Cup the chin with your left hand, taking care that the teeth are together and the tongue safely out of the way. Make sure that the inner part of your hand does not press on the trachea, which would cause the patient discomfort and distress. Turn the head both ways – one is usually more comfortable. Start in the other direction.

Turn the head as far as possible, using considerable traction. Pull both round and up – Grade III in the first direction and up to Grade V in the other.

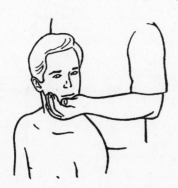

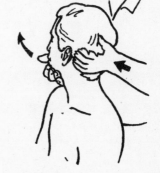

*Figure A1.17*

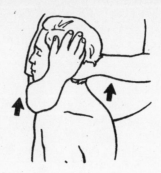

*Figure A1.18*

8. A variation of this can be used for a particularly strong patient. Cradle the chin with your right arm, taking the same precautions as above. Rotate and lift the head steadying the occiput with the left hand. A sharp shrug of the shoulders gives increased thrust.

9. Stand in front of the patient and place a hand on each shoulder. Rotate the patient each way. One way will usually be more

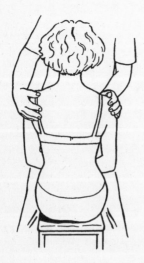

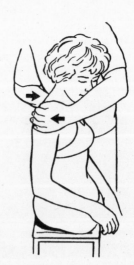

*Figure A1.19*

*Figure A1.20*

comfortable – with pain on the left side, rotating the left shoulder forwards is the more comfortable direction. Now turn the patient in the less comfortable direction as far as possible. The patient relaxes, possibly breathing right out, and receives a thrust in the same direction, Grade III the first side and Grade V the other side.

10. With very strong or tense patients, more leverage is achieved by rotating the patient so that the near shoulder rests as far across your chest as possible. Press the patient firmly towards you so that the shoulder is locked on your chest. Put both hands on the other shoulder and repeat rotation as in number 9.

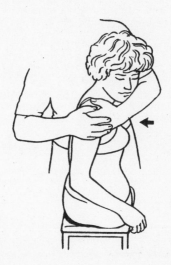

*Figure A1.21*

11. Press your thumb at the base of the neck. Place the other hand so as to assist in pushing the neck firmly sideways. Do the same moving up the neck to the occiput; three presses on either side are often sufficient. Persist with this manoeuvre, even if it is painful. It is particularly effective for headaches.

Use of manoeuvres

- For lumbar pain – number 1 in the region of the spasm from sacrum to mid thoracic spine, numbers 2, 3 and, rarely, 9 or 10.
- For lumbar pain with a tender thoracic spine – as above plus 5 and 6.
- For neck and thoracic pain – numbers 1 and 5 in the thoracic area, 6, 7, 11 and, rarely, 8.
- For neck and headaches – numbers 4, 5 in the high thoracic area, 7, particularly 11 and, rarely, 8.

# APPENDIX

## Action plan for immediate relief of back pain

I am often asked to offer advice over the telephone about how best to manage an acute attack of back pain until treatment is available. As long as your doctor is sure that the pain is caused by back trouble and not by any other illness, there are several things that you can do to help make the pain more endurable, and even to improve the underlying cause.

1. Lying on cushions on the floor, or other suitably hard surface, can bring considerable relief. Try various positions to find the most comfortable.
2. A large cushion placed at the site of the pain helps. The positioning that gives the most relief depends on which groups of muscles are in a cramp. Try putting the cushion under the more painful side.
3. Try to move about, even if it's only to stand up and lie down again. The back gradually seizes up if stationary, so make an effort to move every half an hour or so. As the pain improves, more movement will become possible and relief will be correspondingly faster.
4. When the level of pain permits, try doing the exercises described on pages 266–269. If the pain is in the lower back, the rotational exercise for the lumbar spine will be the most effective. If the pain is in the neck, try the relevant exercise 3. As the condition improves, more of the exercises can be incorporated into your routine.

5. A hot bath can relax the muscles and give considerable relief. Be sure there is someone around to help if the pain is so bad that you cannot get out of the bath unaided.

---

### BEWARE OF A HOT SPOT

Although heat all over the body helps, if it is applied to the painful area alone, it results in an increased arterial circulation at that one place, which causes increased oedema and worsening of the overall situation. This is usually true even if, due to the extra fluid, oxygen and supplies, there seems to be a lessening of the pain in the first instance.

---

6. Chill the area to slow metabolism, which will eventually improve the local tissue circulation. Don't leave an ice-pack on for too long as frostbite may result – a minute is a very rough guide.

   If you have a special cold spray, this should be applied very close to the skin to make a layer of fluid, if possible. A spray will chill the area easily and without mess but is expensive and the substance may be environmentally unfriendly.

7. Massaging the muscles may also be a great help in relaxing them and thus relieving the cramp. It is best done firmly but as far as possible without causing pain. The painful part of the back is often surprisingly unaffected by the immediate pressure of the massage.

8. Take pain-killers, such as soluble aspirin, paracetamol or co-proxamol, which is stronger and may require a doctor's prescription. The recommended maximum dosage of these drugs must not be exceeded, however bad the pain and the desire to alleviate it.

9. Take an anti-inflammatory drug. Most need a doctor's prescription, although Nurofen can be bought from any good chemist and works well.

10. Take a muscle relaxant if you have been prescribed one.

11. An injection of an analgesic such as Marcaine (10ml) can relax the spasm and give immediate relief. Once the injection has worn off, the muscle is quite likely not to go back into a cramp. This will, of course, have to be administered by a doctor.

12. Lastly, there are two things that may give great relief to acute lumbar pain – providing you are an adult of normal or heavy build, not fragile in any way (other than because of the pain) and have had back trouble on and off for several years. If there is a slight member of the family who weighs about five or six stone, with bare feet placed across the vertebrae, he or she can side-step up and down the lumbar and low thoracic vertebrae two or three times.

You will also need help for the second option. Sit on a medium-height stool with your knees together. Your helper should stand in front with his or her legs on each side of your knees. Ask your helper to turn your shoulders as far as possible in the less painful direction and give them a little push. This may well free the back with an almost immediate relief from pain.

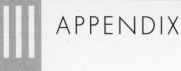

# APPENDIX

## Daily five-minute exercise plan

Regular exercise increases the efficiency of the muscle pump and keeps the muscles in trim. Chronic back pain can be kept at bay with gentle, daily exercise. Everyone has individual requirements in this respect and it is a good idea to develop your own routine, incorporating as many forms of exercise as you (and preferably your doctor) think proper.

The following is, therefore, the barest minimum that will help to keep the back – and only the back – in good working order. Anyone can do these exercises, whether or not you suffer from back problems. Even if you are able to move just a fraction of an inch, they will help increase movement and flexibility, and ultimately reduce pain.

### The neck
1. Turn the head, looking from side to side as far as possible, six times each way.

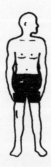

2. Tilt the head from side to side as far as possible, six times each way.

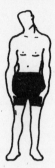

3. Rotate the head, keeping the chin to the front, six times each way.

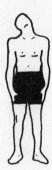

The thoracic area

1. Rotate the shoulder girdle, with the arms hanging down, six times in each direction.

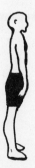

2. Pull the shoulders backwards and forwards as far as possible six times.

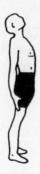

3. Arch the back pushing the shoulders back six times.

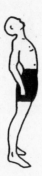

The lumbar spine

1. Rotate the lumbar spine six times with the arms out to the side at about 45 degrees. At the extreme of each movement, give the arms a flick in the same direction to give slight extra movement.

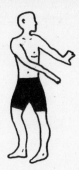

2. Lean over as far as possible first to one side and then the other, six times.

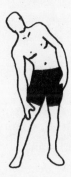

3. Arch the back as far as possible backwards, and then very slightly forwards using the lumbar spine and hips as the pivot. Again do this six times.

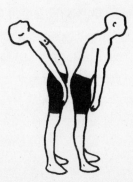

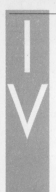

# APPENDIX

## Resuscitation

*Twenty thousand people who become unconscious with a heart attack die each year because they were not given the correct first aid.*
*If a person has a heart attack and becomes unconscious it is important to know what to do.*

## BREATHING

The first thing is to assess if they are still breathing: look for chest movement and feel for breath coming out of the mouth, either with the back of the hand or on your cheek. You will need to spend 4 to 5 seconds to be sure of your decision. If at all possible phone for an ambulance as the first priority, because whatever you do subsequently is only buying time before experts arrive with specialized equipment. If you cannot phone for any reason, call for help to send for an ambulance while you attend to the actual first aid.

If the person is breathing, lay him on his back, put the head to one side and lift the chin to ensure a clear airway. *Make sure that you can feel the air coming in and out of the mouth freely.* Movements of the chest are not enough as a guide because these will take place even if the airway is completely blocked. Pulling the chin up more firmly will usually restore a free airway and it may need continuous lifting to maintain unobstructed breathing (see figure A4.1).

If the breathing should stop at any time, then artificial respiration should be started.

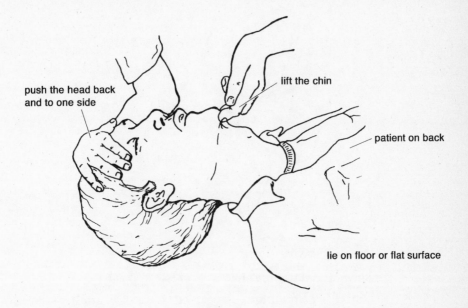

push the head back and to one side

lift the chin

patient on back

lie on floor or flat surface

*Figure A4.1* The airway

## HEARTBEAT

As has been discussed, the heart sends a sudden surge of blood into the arteries which expands them suddenly and this can be felt as a 'pulse' in any artery that can be palpated (felt). The wrist, at the base of the thumb, is the place most commonly used by doctors but the easiest place, especially if the operator is at the head end taking care of the airway, is the large carotid artery which runs up to the head (see figure A4.2). It is very readily found between the voice box and the large neck muscles, just above the collar bone. Practice feeling it on yourself so that you are certain of its exact location.

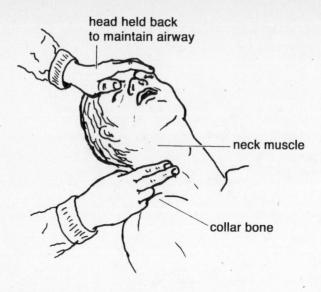

head held back
to maintain airway

neck muscle

collar bone

*Figure A4.2* Carotid pulse.

If the heart is not beating effectively or has stopped, there will be no pulse, and either condition is regarded as cardiac arrest and will normally result in the death of the patient. The casualty may have a good colour at first, but as the blood either drains out of the face he will go pale, or as the oxygen content of the blood becomes used up, the complexion will become blue or grey. The lips have a very thin membrane so the colour is best assessed by looking at them. Prompt, correct measures will save the life of a very large number of these people. If there is cardiac arrest there will be respiratory failure, so first aid must combine artificial respiration with heart compression to maintain a basic oxygenated circulation of the blood, especially to the brain. This is known as cardiopulmonary resuscitation (CPR).

## ARTIFICIAL RESPIRATION

1. Send for an ambulance.
2. Place the patient on the back.
3. Tilt the head well back with your one hand on the forehead.
4. Lift the chin with your other hand but ensure that the mouth is still open.
5. Take a deep breath.
6. Make an airtight joint between yours and the patient's mouth, pinch the patient's nostrils together and breathe out into the patient's lungs steadily over a period of about 2 seconds.
7. Allow the chest to collapse as far as it can.
8. Repeat the process again.
9. If the patient's ribs do not expand as you breathe into his mouth try to improve the airway:

   a) Try pulling the chin up more firmly.

   b) Clear the mouth of any foreign body (dentures etc.).

   c) Try to improve the seal between the two mouths

10. If the patient resumes spontaneous respiration he should be turned onto his side by bending the arm nearest to a right angle and then pulling his opposite arm across his chest. Then grasp the furthest thigh and pull it over toward you, taking the whole body with it as you roll it onto its side.  Keep checking the respiration, pulse and airway. Position the upper knee, thigh and elbow at right angles to prevent the patient from falling right over onto his face (see figure A4.3).

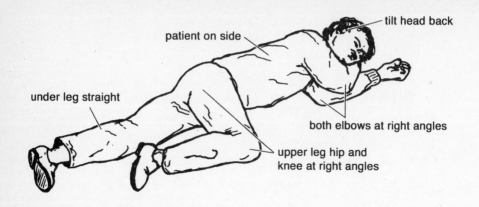

*Figure A4.3* Recovery position.

## CARDIOPULMONARY RESUSCITATION (CPR)

1. Note the exact time. This can be a very valuable piece of inform-ation for the expert team when it arrives.
2. Send for help or get someone else to telephone for an ambulance.
3. Place the patient flat on his back.
4. Give two 'mouth to mouth' exchange breaths.
5. Put the middle finger of one hand in the V where the two sets of ribs meet at the bottom. Put the ball of the other hand's thumb about 5 cms (2 inches) above this, after running it down the breast bone. Then place the first hand on top of the one with the palm over the breast bone and link the fingers (see figure A4.4).
6. Kneel and position yourself directly over the patient's chest with your elbows straight (see figure A4.5).
7. Press very firmly and evenly down, to depress the chest wall by about 5 cms (2 inches) using the 'heel' of the hand – not the fingers. Release the pressure and then repeat the process at as near 80 (almost one and a half to a second) compressions a minute as you can get.

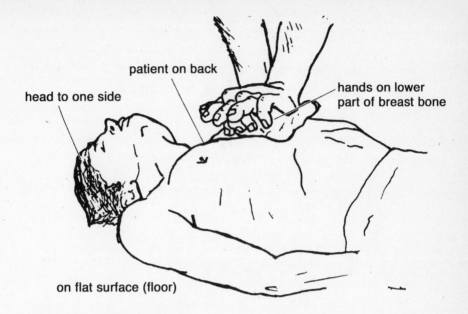

*Figure A4.4* Cardiopulmonary resuscitation.

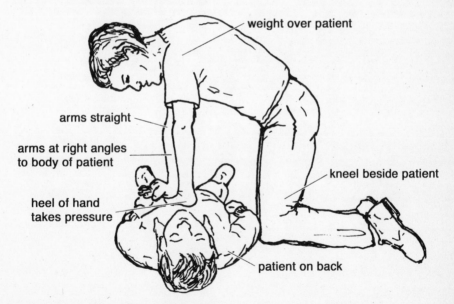

*Figure A4.5* Cardiopulmonary resuscitation.

8. If unaided, give 15 compressions and then two breaths. Keep up this alternation until help arrives or the patient begins to recover.

9. If there is someone to assist, one should give the artificial respiration and the other the cardiac massage, both continuously.

# V APPENDIX

## A note on tonsillectomy

by Mike Dilkes MS, FRCS(Ed), FRCS(Otol), FRCS(ORL)
Medical Director, The London Laser Clinic; Consultant Ear,
Nose and Throat Surgeon, St. Bartholomew's Hospital,
London.

Tonsillectomy is one of the oldest operations in surgery. It has a well-established place in Ear, Nose and Throat practice, with some 85,000 procedures being performed per year in the United Kingdom.

The procedure aims to remove part of the glandular ring of tissue surrounding the throat (Waldeyer's ring). Tonsillectomy generally applies to removal of the 'palatine' tonsils, which sit at the back of the mouth, in the side walls of the throat, near the 'dangly down thing' we surgeons know as the uvula. There are other forms of tonsillectomy, however, in particular lingual tonsillectomy, which treats tonsil tissue at the back of the tongue, although it is not possible to see this tissue on simple inspection.

The indications for tonsillectomy are wide, ranging from recurrent acute tonsillitis, chronic tonsillitis, tonsil stone formation, some causes of halitosis or bad taste in the mouth, quinsy, obstructive sleep apnoea and snoring, to the treatment of psoriasis and other skin conditions.

A number of very large audits have been performed, looking at the success of tonsillectomy in treating conditions such as these. The numbers of patients involved in these audits has been in the tens of thousands. Unequivocally, this operation is very successful in relieving the problems described. There is no good evidence that we might 'miss' our tonsils; instead the evidence shows that they are better removed, particularly if symptoms are troublesome.

Tonsillectomy was first performed in the UK in the nineteenth century, using ether anaesthesia and clumsy tonsil grasping instruments with long, sharp knives for dissection. Cautery of bleeding points was achieved by using red hot irons, or similar devices. Initially, there was a high peri-operative and post-operative mortality and morbidity. With time and the development of better instruments and anaesthesia, this dangerous and unpleasant procedure became increasingly acceptable to the public at large. New techniques, such as guillotine tonsillectomy, were tried, with great success. As medical equipment was developed over the twentieth century, purpose-designed instruments and electrical diathermy (unipolar and bipolar) were introduced, such that the operation generally performed today (dissection tonsillectomy) is unchanged over at least 20 years. Newer techniques, such as cryosurgery, plasma knives and KTP laser have not shown any real advantages over this long-standing and successful procedure.

The problem with the dissection tonsillectomy is that it has not completely circumvented the risk issues surrounding the operation. In particular, post-operative haemorrhage rates remain relatively high (under 10%), and it remains a very painful procedure, with severe soreness in the throat radiating to the ear and jaw for up to three weeks. Generally a considerable amount of time off school or work is required in the convalescent period. These problems relate mainly to teenagers and adults. Children, particularly when under the age of seven, tend to suffer relatively little after tonsillectomy.

Recently, a new technique has evolved in the UK, in which a pre-existing technique in the USA (laser tonsillotomy) has been developed and improved, incorporating experienced gained from a new laser cancer technique in Germany (Steiner surgery). This new technique involves a high powered carbon dioxide laser, used in SwiftlaseTM mode with an operating microscope and a micromanipulator. The principle is that the tonsil is vapourised from its inside surface towards its outside, in a carefully controlled, bloodless manner. This is markedly different from the standard dissection tonsillectomy, in which the tonsil is removed by dissecting around the outside of the tissue, where the blood vessels and muscle of the throat lies. Exposure of these structures leads to the bleeding risk and the pain, since the revealed muscle ulcerates when in contact with saliva and its enzymes. Because of the large area exposed, healing is slow (it heals by 'secondary intention'). Thus, the laser vapourisation technique removes tonsil tissue to the edge of its capsule, but does not go through it. Since the muscle and blood vessels lie beyond the capsule, they are not affected. Since only the capsule and a thin rim of tonsil tissue is left behind after this procedure, little ulceration and pain occur, the blood vessel layer is not entered, and therefore this is not a problem with respect to bleeding. However, the vast majority of active tonsil tissue will have been removed, thus the patient's symptoms after surgery are very well treated, without the suffering incurred when undergoing the standard technique.

Our results, in nearly 200 patients treated, confirm that pain and bleeding after tonsillectomy is much reduced when compared to standard techniques. Recurrence of significant tonsil symptoms after treatment occurs approximately 1% of the time – the same as with standard dissection tonsillectomy.

# GLOSSARY

Abdominal migraine Episodic attacks of abdominal pain.

Abraham's box A box that cures or controls illness by correcting faulty waves of radiation produced by the body.

Acupressure Also called shiatsu. Acupuncture points treated by finger pressure.

Acute Severe and sudden symptoms, that have a quick resolution one way or the other.

Adrenalin Hormone that largely mimics the action of the sympathetic nerves.

Alveoli Air cells in the lungs.

Alexander technique Retraining the body to eliminate acquired postural faults.

Allergy Super-sensitive reaction to certain substances and stimuli.

Analgesic Pain-killer.

Angina Pain.

Angina pectoris Pain in the chest – heart pain.

Ankylosing spondylitis Disease that causes both spine and hip joints to become stiff.

Anti-allergics Drugs to counteract allergies.

Anti-inflammatory drugs Given to counteract inflammation.

Antibody Substance produced by the body in response to antigens, which usually take the form of bacteria or viruses.

Aorta Large artery leading from the heart.

Aromatherapy Complementary therapy using essential oils.

Arteriole Very small artery.

Artery Vessel that takes blood from the heart around the body.

Arteriosclerosis Degenerative condition of the arteries.

Atrio-ventricular node (AV) Special conducting material in the heart.

Arthritis Inflammation of a joint. There are many different causes.

Atherosclerosis Nodules of arteriosclerosis.

Atrium auricle Thin-walled entrance cavities of the heart.

Beta-blockers Substances that block the action of the sympathetic nerve system.

Brain stem The part of the brain where the nerves come out.

Candida Yeast that infests the body causing thrush.

Capillaries Minute vessels that join arteries to veins and transmit oxygen and nutrients to the tissues, removing carbon dioxide and waste from them.

Carbon dioxide Gas resulting from tissue activity, released when we exhale.

Carotid artery Large artery in the neck supplying the head.

Carpal tunnel syndrome Nerve pinched in the wrist causing pain, numbness and loss of strength.

Cerebellum Little brain at the base of the skull that controls automatic repetitive actions.

Cerebral To do with the brain.

Chiropractic Manipulating misaligned bones to restore health.

Cholesterol A variety of alcohol found in the bile, blood and all cells. It is a constituent of cell membranes, hormones, bile acids, sex hormones and vitamin D.

Chronic Disease lasting over a long period of time.

Clot A semi-solid mass produced by coagulation of blood.

Coccyx End bones of the spine forming the residual tail.

Collateral circulation Blood vessels running parallel to one that is damaged.

Congenital A condition with which you are born.

Cortisone Hormone secreted by the adrenal gland cortex.

Congestive heart failure A gradual failure of the heart when fluid collects because the heart is unable to pump it away fast enough.

Coronary heart disease Disease in the blood vessels that supply the heart.

Coronary thrombosis A blockage in an artery that supplies the heart muscle.

Coronary artery An artery that supplies the heart muscle.

Cramp Painful involuntary contraction of a muscle.

Depression A medical condition the main symptoms of which are inertia, fatigue and sleeplessness.

Diabetes Insufficient insulin resulting in damaging levels of free sugar.

Diastolic The period from the end of one heart contraction to the start of the next. Hence the lowest pressure level of the blood.

Digitalis The dried leaf of the purple foxglove used to treat heart failure.

Dilating Increasing internal diameter.

Duodenum First 12 inches of the small intestine.

Electro-cardiogram (ECG) An electrical tracing of the impulses from the heart muscles.

Elimination diet A diet that eliminates various foods and reintroduces them one by one to discover a food intolerance.

Encephalon Brain.

Endorphins Chemical transmitters that control pain and other functions.

ESR test A blood test to check for the activity of certain diseases.

Facet joints In the back, the joints between one vertebral arch and another. The term applies to a number of joints in the body.

Faradism An interrupted electrical current used to stimulate nerves.

Femoral nerve A large nerve running down the front of the thigh.

Fibrositis **Non-joint rheumatic (or other) pain.**

Flexion **Bending a joint to approximate its parts.**

Frozen shoulder **A condition in which the shoulder joint becomes stiff and very painful.**

Ganglion **Virtually a small brain. There are many of these nerve centres scattered about the body.**

Golfer's elbow **A painful elbow due to a torn muscle.**

Hiatus hernia **The stomach bulges into the chest through an enlarged hole in the diaphragm.**

Homoeopathy **Treatment of disease by taking minute doses of substances that produce the symptoms, thus activating the body's immune system.**

HDL/LDL **High and low density lipids, which carry cholesterol to the tissues.**

Hormones **Chemical messengers that affect distant tissues.**

HRT **Hormone replacement therapy for women after the menopause.**

Humidity **Increased water in the atmosphere, sometimes said to make rheumatism worse.**

Hydrotherapy **Therapeutic treatment with water.**

Hypertension **High blood pressure.**

Hyposympathetic tone (HST) **Reduced activity of the sympathetic system, causing illness.**

Hypoglycaemic **Low blood sugar.**

Intermittent claudication **A disease of arteries in which they cut off the blood supply at times, usually causing pain in the calf muscles.**

Intervertebral discs **Flexible, elastic pads separating the vertebrae from each other.**

Ionization **The forming of an electrical charge on an atom by adding or subtracting electrons.**

Ligament **Strong, fibrous support connecting bones across joints.**

Lipoprotein **Complexes of lipids and proteins that have many properties of proteins.**

Lumbar The lower part of the back, between the thoracic spine and the sacrum.

Lumbar curve The normal curve of the lumbar spine that gives it flexibility.

Lumbar sympathetic ganglia The nerve activity centres in the lumbar region.

Lumbo-sacral joint The joint between the spine and the sacrum.

Lymph ducts Tubes that carry lymph from the tissue spaces to the lymph nodes and then back to the veins. The sewers of the body.

Lymph nodes The waste disposal units in the lymphatic sewage system.

Magnesium A trace metal the shortage of which in red blood cells causes tiredness.

Manipulation A sharp thrust to move a joint further than it could previously go.

Menopause The cessation of menstruation.

Migraine Very severe, one-sided, sick headache.

Motor nerves Nerves that transmit impulses from the brain to the muscles.

Moxa A herb used to stimulate acupuncture trigger points, or to heat the end of an acupuncture needle, enhancing its effect.

Muscle pump The squeezing effect of a contracting muscle, sending blood via the veins to the heart.

Myalgia Painful muscles.

Myocardium Heart muscle.

Myalgic encephalomyelitis (ME) Also known as post-viral syndrome and chronic fatigue syndrome. Symptoms include extreme tiredness.

Naturopathy Treating illness with diet, exercise, hydrotherapy and osteopathy.

Nerve root Part of the nerve that goes from the spinal cord through the neural canal in the backbone to form a peripheral nerve.

Neural canal Space formed between vertebrae through which the nerves pass.

NSAIDs (non-steroidal anti-inflammatory drugs) Drugs that do not contain cortisone.

Occiput The back of the skull.

Occlusion Blockage.

Oedema Excessive fluid in the tissues, causing swelling.

Oesophagus Tube extending from the mouth to the stomach.

Oestrins Female hormones.

Oestrogen Any substance that mimics the action of the ovarian hormone Oestradiol.

Osmosis Force that draws fluid through a permeable membrane.

Osteopathy Manipulative treatment of joints and soft tissues.

Osteoporosis Thinning and weakening of the bones, mainly present in post-menopausal women.

Pacemaker The sino-atrial node that controls the rate of the heart; an electronic gadget inserted to set the pace of the heart after its own control has failed.

Paget's disease A thickening of certain bones in the body, notably the skull.

Palpation To examine the body with the hands, relying on sense of touch.

Parasympathetic nervous system The nerve chain that controls digestion.

Paravertebral At the side of a vertebra.

Pelvis Several bones joined together to form a basin at the base of the abdomen.

Peptic ulcer An ulcer of the membrane lining the stomach or duodenum.

Physical medicine Treatment by physical means – massage, manipulation, electricity, the application of heat or cold.

Physiology The study of the workings of the body.

Physiotherapy Remedial exercises; also some forms of physical medicine.

Plaque A flat area, a patch.

Plasma The fluid part of the blood in which the corpuscles are suspended.

Platelets Flat cells in the blood needed for clotting to take place.

Polymyalgia **Pain affecting a number of muscles.**

Post-viral syndrome **Also called ME (myalgic encephalomyelitis). An illness with many symptoms, the main one being tiredness.**

Prostaglandins **Chemical messengers in the body that have a wide range of effects, including enhancing the inflammatory process.**

Psychological **To do with the mind or mental activity.**

Psychosomatic **A physical symptom caused or aggravated by psychological stress.**

Pulse **A wave of expansion down the arteries caused by the sudden increase of the blood pressure as the heart beats.**

Pyloric sphincter **A circular band of muscle that controls the exit from the stomach.**

Quiescent **Symptomless – the illness may be inactive or dormant.**

Raynaud's disease **Arterial disease that causes an extreme reaction to cold, especially in the hands and feet.**

Red cells **Cells that transport oxygen and carbon dioxide in the blood.**

Referred pain **Pain felt in a part of the body other than where it originates.**

Reflexology **The manipulation and massage of specific areas of the hands and feet that affect particular areas of the body.**

Sacrum **Five fused vertebrae in the lower back that form part of the pelvic basin.**

Sciatica **Shooting pain down the sciatic nerve in the back of the leg.**

Sciatic nerve **Large sensory and motor nerve that runs down the back of the leg.**

Sclerosing agent **A substance that hardens the tissues.**

Sensor **An organ located at the beginning of a nerve. Each one has a special function, such as perceiving cold, heat, pain or vibration.**

Serotonin **Chemical messenger in the body.**

Shiatsu **Also called acupressure. Acupuncture points treated by finger pressure.**

Sino-atrial node Also known as the sino-auricular node. The main timekeeper of the heart, sited in the right atrium, with a natural beat of between 60 and 100 per minute.

Spasm An involuntary protective muscle contraction, controlled through the nervous system and therefore symptomless.

Sphincter A ring of muscle that closes a tube or orifice.

Spinal cord Huge nerve complex that passes down the neural canal formed by the vertebrae. An extension of the brain.

Splanchnic ganglion A group of nerve centres influencing the bowel.

Spondylitis An active inflammatory process in the spinal joints.

Spondylolisthesis A condition in which one vertebra slips forward on to another.

Spondylosis A degenerative condition of the vertebral joints.

Square-wave pulse A form of faradism.

Stellate ganglion A group of sympathetic nerve centres located at the base of the neck that controls a number of functions and organs, including the heart.

Sterno-mastoid muscle Large muscle in the neck, attached to the base of the skull.

Steroids A group of chemicals derived from cholesterol, including sex hormones, cardiac glycosides, hormones and vitamin D.

Subconscious An active part of the brain that functions unnoticed.

Surged faradism An interrupted electrical current that has a rhythmic change of intensity. When applied to a nerve, it produces alternating contractions and relaxation in the relevant muscle.

Sympathetic nerve chain An interconnected line of little brains that process the activity of the sympathetic nervous system. They maintain most body parameters and with adrenalin put the body in a supreme state of activity in an emergency.

Syndrome A group of symptoms and signs that constitute a definite disease.

Systolic The period when the heart contracts, having the higher of the two blood pressure readings.

Tendon The wire-like part of a muscle that joins it to a bone.

Tennis elbow Painful condition of the elbow, caused by a torn muscle.

TENS (transcutaneous electrical nerve stimulation) Electrical impulses applied to the skin via small pads to relieve pain.

Testosterone A steroid, a male sex hormone.

Thoracic To do with the chest.

Thoracic curve The curve in the thoracic spine that enables it to absorb stress or a blow.

Thorax The part of the trunk between the neck and the abdomen.

Thrombus A blood clot formed in, and remaining in, a blood vessel.

Tissue fluid Fluid that has left the blood in the capillaries and is bathing the cells.

Tissue space The space between the tissue cells where the tissue fluid circulates.

Trachea The windpipe.

Traction Forceable pulling apart of the vertebrae (or other structures).

Ultrasonic waves Very high frequency sound waves, far above the hearing limits of the human ear.

Vagus nerve The main parasympathetic outlet.

Valve (heart) An organ that allows blood to flow out of the heart, preventing it from regurgitating back to the chambers or blood vessels.

Veins Blood vessels that carry blood from the capillaries to the heart.

Ventricle (heart) The two main pumping chambers of the heart.

Ventricular fibrillation Uncoordinated, ineffective contractions of the ventricles.

Venule Minute vein.

Vertebrae Bones that together make up the spine.

Virus Micro-organism that survives in a host's living cell.

White cells **Disease-fighting soldiers of the body. Found in the blood and lymphatic system, they are the basis for the immune system.**

Yoga **System of exercises that increases the life force and flexibility.**

# USEFUL ADDRESSES

BackCare (formerly the National Back Pain Association)
16 Elmtree Road
Teddington
Middlesex TW11 8ST
Tel: 020 8977 5474
Website: *www.backpain.org*

Help the Aged
207-221 Pentonville Road
London N1 9UZ
Tel: 020 7278 1114
Email: *info@helptheaged.org.uk*

The Institute for Complementary Medicine
PO Box 194
London SE16 7QZ
Tel: 020 7237 5165
Email: *info@icmedicine.co.uk*

The ME (Myalgic Encephalomyelitis) Association
4 Top Angel
Buckingham Industrial Park
Buckingham
Buckinghamshire MK18 1TH
Tel: 0871 222 7824
Website: *www.meassociation.org.uk*

Migraine Action Association
Unit 6, Oakley Hay Lodge Business Park
Great Folds Road
Great Oakley
Northants NN18 9AS
Tel: 01536 461333
Email: *info@migraine.org.uk*

National Ankylosing Spondylitis Society
PO Box 179
Mayfield
East Sussex TN20 6ZL
Tel: 01435 873527
Email: *nass@nass.co.uk*

Research Council for Complementary Medicine
27a Devonshire Street
London W1G 6PN
Tel: 020 7935 7499
Email: *info@rccm.org.uk*

Society of Teachers of the Alexander Technique
1st Floor
Linton House
39-51 Highgate Road
London NW5 1RS
Tel: 0845 230 7828
Email: *enquiries@stat.org.uk*

Yoga for Health Foundation
Ickwell Bury
Northill
Biggleswade
Bedfordshire SG18 9EF
Tel: 01767 627271
Email: *admin@yogaforhealthfoundation.co.uk*

# INDEX

abdominal migraine 164–5, 280
Abraham's box 234–5, 280
acid 159–60, 161, 164
acupressure 235–6, 280
acute 280
adrenalin 101, 280
ageing 22–3
  definition 23
  difference with degeneration 23
Alexander technique 237, 280
allergy 59–60, 108–9, 127–9, 280
alveoli 280
analgesics 227, 280
  co-proxamol (distalgesic) 227
  dihydrocodeine (DF118) 227
  morphine, phenazocine, methadone 227
  paracetamol 227
angina 189, 190–1, 280
Ankylosing spondylitis 280
anti-allergics 127, 280
anti-inflammatory drugs 61, 63, 64, 172, 227, 280
  non-steroidal 228–9
  steroids 228
antibody 10, 40, 281
anxiety/fright 110, 161
aorta 178, 281
aromatherapy 237–8, 281
arteriole 10, 35, 281
arteriosclerosis 281
artery 10, 281
  blocked by clot 193
  disease 174
  narrowed by disease in its wall 191–2
  narrowed by nerve control 189
  spasm 192–3
arthritis 62, 112, 130, 281
  hip joint 166–7
    helpful treatment 172
    misleading distribution of pain 168–70
    missed diagnosis 167–70

    pain lies in hip joint 170–1
    pain in lumbar region 170
    pain referred from back 171
    patient knows best 170–1
    X-rays 168
  shoulder/hand 146–8
    emergency action 149–52
atherosclerosis 191–2, 281
atrio-ventricular node (AV) 184, 281
atrium auricle 281

back strain relief
  beds 246
  loss of weight 247
  massage rollers/vibrating pads, seat lumbar supportsback strain relief 247–8
  shoes 248
  working surfaces 248
beta-blockers 209–10, 281
blood circulation 10–13, 14, 35–6, 118–19, 202
blood pressure 107, 183
brain stem 104, 281
bruising 29–30, 207, 217–18
  treating 219–21
buttock pain 169–70, 171

calcium 58, 61, 63, 229
calf pain 77–9
candida 129–30, 281
capillaries 10–12, 36, 281
carbon dioxide 10, 281
cardio-pulmonary resuscitation (CPR) 185, 274–6
carotid artery 281
carpal tunnel syndrome 155–6, 281
central nervous system 98
centre of spine pain 74
cerebellum 8, 281
cerebral 281
cervical tensional headache 146
chiropractic 281

chiropractors 20, 234
cholesterol 281
chronic/recurring pain
  confusion/controversy surrounding
    19–20
  five forms of illness 21–8
  old injuries 20–1
  onset of pain 39
    complete rest 39
    muscular effort 39
    posture 41
    stretching the muscle 41
    tonsils 40–1
    viral infection 39–40
  reaching crisis point 41–2
  shocks to the system 28–9
    lack of symptoms 32–5
    nature's response 29–32
    results of 29
  signs leading to attack 35–6
    building up to critical level 36–9
chronis 281
clot 282
coccyx 3, 282
coffee 128
collateral circulation 282
compensation 35
congestive heart failure 282
coronary heart disease 177–8, 282
  acute disease 184–5
  aids to recovery
    normal lifestyle 211–12
    positive attitude of mind 210–11
    support from family/friends 213–14
  causes of blockage 188–9
    arterial spasm 192–3
    artery narrowed by disease in its wall
      191–2
    artery narrowed by nerve control
      189–91
    clots 193
  chronic disease 182
    congestive failure 182
    diminishing elasticity of arterial walls
      183
    rapid failure 182
    valve disorders 183
  coronary arteries 178–80, 282
    importance of resuscitation 185–6
    malfunction of stellate ganglion 193–7
    management of problem 207–9
      beta-blockers 209–10
    problems 180–5
    questions concerning 176–7

    attacks in early morning 202
    coronary/cerebral arteries at fault 200
      gender differences 206
      myocardial infarct precedes
        thrombosis 202–3
      no known risk factors 206
      peak ages 205
      playing squash/jogging 204–5
      tests/ECG as normal 199–200
      transient dizzy spells 203–4
      unwell for several days 198–9
      well periods between attacks 201
    reaching crisis point
      anxiety/worry 196
      complete rest 196
      smoking 197
      unaccustomed exercise 196
      weather 196–7
    severity of spasm 197
      amount that spasm narrows artery
        197
      degree/activity of disease in artery 197
      duration of spasm 197
    symptoms 214–15
      aches 215
      extreme tiredness 215
      indigestion, headachs, dizzy spells
        215–16
    triggers of attack
      blockage of blood supply 186
      failure of muscles through toxic
        interference 187
      other factors 188
      sudden disruption of transmitting
        mechanism 187
cortisol 124
cortisone 62, 128, 228, 282
cramp 43–4, 58–9, 63, 169–70

depression 110, 132–3, 165–6, 282
diabetes 282
diaphragm 162
diastolic 282
diazepam (Valium) 229
diet/food 59–60, 129, 133, 159–60, 188,
  238
digitalis 182, 282
dilating 282
disc problems 80–2
drugs
  analgesics 227
  anti-inflammatory 227–9
  application of cold 230
  muscle relaxants 229

duodenal ulcer 161–2
duodenum 159, 160, 282

electro-cardiogram (ECG) 176, 199, 202,
    204, 282
elimination diet 282
encephalon 282
endorphins 282
ESR (erythrocyte sedimentation rate) test
    114, 282
exercise 187, 196, 206, 239, 265–9

facet joints 6–7, 74–7, 87, 97, 169, 207,
    282
faradism 64, 221–3, 249–50, 282, 287
fatigue see tiredness
femoral nerve 168, 282
fibrositis 112, 283
fight-or-flight reactions 52, 101–2, 103
flatulence 159–60
flexion 29, 283
food see diet/food
frozen shoulder 153, 283

ganglion 98, 104, 136, 283
    lumbar sympathetic 166–74
    splanchnic 158–66
    stellate 137–57, 175
gastric ulcer 160–2
golfer's elbow 283
Golgi tendon organs 27–8

HDL/IDL 283
headache see cervical tensional headache;
    migraine
heart attacks see coronary heart disease
heel pain 77–9
hiatus hernia 162–4, 283
hip pain 167–72
homeopathy 240, 283
hormones 61, 283
HRT (hormone replacement therapy)
    61–2, 206, 283
humidity 57, 283
hydrotherapy 240–1, 283
hypertension 183, 283
hypoglycaemic 107, 283
hyposympathetic tone (HST) 84, 90–4,
    105, 283
    compensatory reactions of the brain
        depression 110
        inability to cope with change in
            routine 110–13
        sleep inversion 110

tense state of mind 110
tension 109–10
low sympathetic drive
    extreme tiredness 105–7
    low blood pressure 107
    low blood sugar 107
other back-related diseases 113
parasympathetic over activity
    allergic reaction 108–9
    indigestion 107–8, 127
    putting on weight 108
hyposympathetic tone syndrome (HST)
    136

Icelandic disease see myalgic
    encephalomyelitis (ME)
illness
    five forms 21
        congenital 282
        congenital problems 21
        degenerative conditions 22–4
        infections 21–2
        injury 24–8
        tumours/growths 22
indigestion 107–8, 113, 127, 136, 159,
    159–60
interferential treatment 222
intermittent claudication 174, 283
intervertebral discs 5–6, 79–80, 87, 283
ionization 57, 196–7, 283

knee pain 173–4

leg pain 174
ligaments 13, 15, 219, 283
lipoprotein 283
liquorice sweets 124
lower back pain 72
    sacro-iliac joints 72–3
lumbar 284
    pain 67
        causes of 'click' 67–70
        relief as temporary 71–2
lumbar curve 284
lumbar sympathetic ganglia 166, 284
    arterial diseases in legs 174
    malfunctions
        arthritis of hip joint 166–72
        arthritis of the knee 173–4
lumbar-sacral joint 284
lymph ducts 118–19, 284
lymph nodes 117–19, 122, 123, 284

magnesium 58, 126, 229, 284

Maitland system 241–2
manipulation 223–4, 241–4, 250–62, 284
massage 225, 233
menopause 61, 284
menstruation *see* periods
migraine 113, 137–8, 194, 284
  abdominal 164–5
  causes 138–42
    after chopping wood 145
    after a long car journey 144
    after a night's rest 142
    food 143–4
    getting excited 142–3
    psychological disease 145–6
    on a sunny day 143
mineral deficiency 127, 229
motor nerves 284
Moxa 236, 284
MRI (magnetic resonance imaging) scans
  82–3
muscle pump 10, 13, 14, 171, 284
  poor function 97–8
    central nervous system 98
    parasympathetic nervous system
      98–105
    sympathetic nervous system 98, 100–5
muscle spasms 30–2, 36, 38–9, 43, 97, 219,
  287
  heart attacks 107, 192–3, 207
  leg 172
  spinal injury 136
  treating 219–23
  ulcers 162
  uterus 90
myalgia 114, 284
myalgic encephalomyelitis (ME) 114, 284
  confusion concerning 115–16
  positive approach
    ask specific questions 134–5
    contact relevant association 134
    keep as fit as possible 133
    massage neck/back 134
    modify diet 133
    replace mercury fillings in teeth 134
    replace trace elements 133–4
    take a cold bath every morning 134
  *see also* post-viral syndrome
myocardium 284

naturopathy 242, 284
neck pain 73–4, 112
nerve root 284
neural canal 6–7, 224, 284
neural tethering 224

noradrenaline 124
NSAIDS (non-steroidal anti-inflammatory
  drugs) 228–9, 284

occiput 285
occlusion 285
oedema 36, 38, 43, 136, 210, 219, 231, 285
oesophagus tube 159, 160, 164, 285
oestrins 61, 285
oestrogen 285
orthopaedics 247
osmosis 285
osteopathy 20, 234, 242–3, 285
osteoporosis 61–2, 285
oxygen 178, 188, 190–1

pacemaker 285
Paget's disease 285
palpation 285
parasympathetic nervous system 87, 92,
  98–9, 160, 285
  balance upset by muscle spasm 104–5
  heart attacks 189, 195
paravertebral 112, 285
pelvis 285
peptic ulcer 285
periods (menstruation)
  amenorrhoea 92
  dysmenorrhoea 165
  painful 90
physical medicine 285
physiology 27, 285
physiotherapy 234, 285
pituitary gland 123–4
plaque 285
plasma 11, 285
platelets 285
polymyalgia 286
post-viral syndrome 114, 117–22, 286
  causes 116–17
  lymph nodes 117–22
  sore throat/tonsilities 119–21
  symptoms
    candida infestation 129–30
    complete exhaustion 122–6
    depression 132–3
    food allergy 127–9
    indigestion 127
    poor memory/woolly feeling in the
      head 126
    vitamin/mineral deficiencies 127
    weakness of the joints 130–2
  *see also* low sympathetic drive; myalgic
    encephalomyelitis (ME)

posture 8–9, 48–51
power-assisted micro-manipulation (PAM)
    225
prostaglandins 228, 286
psychological 286
pulse 286
pyloric sphincter 286

quiescent 286

Raynaud's disease 156–8, 194, 286
recurring pain see chronic/recurring pain
red cells 286
referred pain 74, 286
    calf/heel 77–9
    disc problems 80–2
    facet joints 74–7
    intervertebral disc 79–80
    MRI scans 82–3
    spinal stenosis 79
reflexology 245, 286
remobilization 224, 241–4, 250–62
resuscitation 185–6
    artificial respiration 273–4
    breathing 270–1
    cardiopulmonary resuscitation (CPR)
        2746
    heartbeat 271–2
Royal Free disease see myalgic
        encephalomyelitis (ME)

sacro-iliac joints 15–16
sacrum 286
salcitonin 62
salt 59
sciatic nerve 168–9, 286
sciatica 168–9, 286
sclerosing agent 241, 286
sensors 27–8
serotonin 56, 196, 286
sex
    interruption of nerve supply 87
        acute sensitivity 89–90
        blood vessels do not dilate 87–8
        little sensation 88
    low sympathetic drive 90–2
        loss of libido 92–4
    male problems 85–7
shiatsu 286
shoulder pain 73–4
silent back trouble 96–7
sino-atrial node 287
sleep see tiredness
smoking 197

sore throat 119–21
spasms see muscle spasms
sphincter 159–60, 287
spinal column
    circulation of blood 10–13, 14
    description 16–17
    ood design 17–18
    ligaments 13, 15
    maintenance of posture 8–9
    mobility 2
    movement 7–8
    neural canal 6–7
    protection 1–2
    sacro-iliac joints 15–16
    structure 3
        facet joints 6–7
        intervertebral discs 5–6
        spinal muscles 7
        vertebrae 3–4, 16, 24
    support 1
    vertebrae 3–4, 51
spinal cord 287
spinal stenosis 79
splanchnic ganglion 158, 287
    malfunctions
        abdominal migraine 164–5
        depression/other troubles 165–6
        gastric/duodenal ulcers 160–2
        hiatus hernia 162–4
        indigestion/flatulence 159–60
spondylosthesis 287
square-wave pulse 221, 287
stellate ganglion 287
    malfunctions
        arthritis of shoulder/hand 146–52
        carpal tunnel syndrome 155–6
        frozen shoulder 152
        heart disease 175, 193–7
        migraine 137–46
        Raynaud's disease 156–7
        tennis elbow 152–5
sterno-mastoid muscle 287
steroids 228, 287
subconscious 287
surged faradism see faradism
sympathetic drive 159–60
sympathetic nerve chain 52, 287
sympathetic nervous system 98, 100–2,
        107, 132
    heart attacks 192, 199, 202, 204
    (post-)viral infections 117–22
    tug-of-war situation 102–4, 189
syndrome 287
systolic 288

tendon 288
tennis elbow 153–5, 288
TENS (transcutaneous electrical nerve
    stimulation) 236, 288
tension 109–10, 161
testosterone 288
theory/explanation
    bad posture 48–51
    benefits of exercise 44–5
    effect of age 45–6
    ffect of anxiety 51–3
    effect of menopause 61
    effect of pregnancy 62–4
    effect of weather 56–7
    food allergy 59–60
    level of fitness 46–7
    pain after long journey 47–8
    pain at rest after energetic movement 44
    pain in the morning 43–4
    pain as psychosomatic 53–5
    pain/diet relationship 58–9
    viral infections 60–1
    weight/height influences 57–8
thoracic 50, 112, 158, 288
thoracic curve 50, 288
thorax 288
thrombus 192–3, 288
thyroxin 125–6
tiredness 105–7, 110, 122–6, 128
tissue fluid 11, 44, 97–105, 219, 230, 288
tissue space 12, 43, 219, 230, 288
tonsilitis 119–21, 173–4
    procedure 277–9
toxins 173
trachea 288
traction 245, 288
treatment
    Abraham's box 234–5
    acupressure/shiatsu 235
    acupuncture 235–6
    Alexander technique 237
    aromatherapy 237–8
    basic problem 218–19
    bed rest 238
    clinical nutrition 238
    corsets, collars, plaster–casts 238–9
    drugs 226–30
    exercise 239
    faith, spiritual, natural healing 239–40
    homeopathy 240

    hydrotherapy 240–1
    immediate relief 263–5
    injections of sclerosing agents 241
    manipulation 223–4, 241–4
    massage 225
    medical herbalism 244
    meditation 245
    over-riding nature's cure 219–21
    power-assisted micro-manipulation
        (PAM) 225
    questions answered
        age of patient 233–4
        feeling ill afterwards 232–3
        length of treatment 230–1
        location of treatment 234
        pain of treatment 232
        trouble over many years 231–2
    reflexology 245
    remobilization 224, 241–4
    surged faradism 221–3
    surgery 245
    traction 245–6
    ultrasonic waves 225–6
    yoga 246

ulcers 160–2
ultrasonic waves 64, 174, 221, 225–6, 250,
    288
underlying problems 84

vagus nerve 98, 101, 104–5, 159, 160,
    288
valve (heart) 183, 288
veins 13, 288
ventricle (heart) 288
ventricular fibrillation 185, 288
venule 288
vertebrae 3–4, 51, 288
viral infection 121–2
virus 60–1, 119, 288
vitamin deficiency 127, 133–4

weather 57, 196–7
weight-gain 108
white cells 289
working in partnership 66

X-rays 23–4, 168

yoga 246, 289